T0214726

SpringerBriefs in Statistics

SpringerBriefs present concise summaries of cutting-edge research and practical applications across a wide spectrum of fields. Featuring compact volumes of 50 to 125 pages, the series covers a range of content from professional to academic. Typical topics might include:

- A timely report of state-of-the art analytical techniques
- A bridge between new research results, as published in journal articles, and a contextual literature review
- A snapshot of a hot or emerging topic
- An in-depth case study or clinical example
- A presentation of core concepts that students must understand in order to make independent contributions

SpringerBriefs in Statistics showcase emerging theory, empirical research, and practical application in Statistics from a global author community.

SpringerBriefs are characterized by fast, global electronic dissemination, standard publishing contracts, standardized manuscript preparation and formatting guidelines, and expedited production schedules.

Marcel van Oijen • Mark Brewer

Probabilistic Risk Analysis and Bayesian Decision Theory

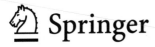 Springer

Marcel van Oijen
Edinburgh, UK

Mark Brewer
BioSS Office, The James Hutton Institute
Aberdeen, UK

ISSN 2191-544X   ISSN 2191-5458   (electronic)
SpringerBriefs in Statistics
ISBN 978-3-031-16332-6   ISBN 978-3-031-16333-3   (eBook)
https://doi.org/10.1007/978-3-031-16333-3

This Springer imprint is published by the registered company Springer Nature Switzerland AG
The registered company address is: Gewerbestrasse 11, 6330 Cham, Switzerland

Preface

Why This Book?

Risk analysis is often the first step before decision-making. But what is risk, and how can we rigorously analyse it? How do we quantify the key components of risk? There is considerable confusion about these questions in the academic literature, and this book is our attempt to provide answers. We aim to provide clear definitions, formulas and algorithms.

Risk involves a stress factor or hazard and a system that is vulnerable to that hazard. The risk is high when both hazard probability and system vulnerability are high. These ideas are expressed in an influential United Nations report on disaster management (UN, 1992) which defined risk as "expected losses" to be calculated as "the product of hazard and vulnerability." Likewise, the Intergovernmental Panel on Climate Change (IPCC, 2014) represented risk as "the probability of occurrence of hazardous events or trends multiplied by the impacts if these events or trends occur." These definitions make intuitive sense, but they need to be formalised to make risk analysis unambiguous and uniquely quantifiable. Unfortunately, the literature has been deficient in that respect, with especially the definition of vulnerability lacking any consensus (Ionescu et al., 2009).

In earlier work, we showed how risk, hazard probability and system vulnerability should be defined to allow formal decomposition of risk as the mathematical product of the other two terms (Van Oijen et al., 2013). We applied this risk decomposition to the problem of present and future drought risk of vegetation across Europe (Van Oijen et al., 2014). We also applied the method to forest data sets and introduced formulas for quantifying uncertainties associated with sampling-based estimates of risk and its two components (Van Oijen and Zavala, 2019). These studies form a useful basis for rigorous probabilistic risk analysis that is slowly becoming adopted more widely (e.g. Kuhnert et al., 2017, Zhou et al., 2018, He et al., 2021, and Nandintsetseg et al., 2021). However, the applications have so far been restricted to 2-factor sampling-based risk analysis. This book expands the approach to a comprehensive theory of risk analysis and elucidates the links with Bayesian decision theory. We derive formulas for estimating risk and its components, and for quantifying the uncertainties associated with all terms. Computer code is shown as well and the R-files may be downloaded from the link available in chapter footnotes.

Who Is this Book for?

This book is intended for researchers and decision-makers with an interest in rigorous risk analysis. Some familiarity with probability theory will make the book easier to digest, but the book does contain simple introductions to both probabilistic risk analysis (PRA) and Bayesian decision theory (BDT). We have tried to avoid jargon and define all terms that we use in the book itself.

To show the practical use of the theory, we included many examples of applications, mostly using very simple artificial data sets. The examples are taken from the fields of the environmental sciences, including ecology and forestry, but our analytical methods are completely generic. We hope that those from other fields will find inspiration for application in their own work. The theory is applicable to both discrete event hazards (e.g. earthquakes) and continuous hazards (e.g. pollution that is never zero or water availability that is never optimal).

Notation

The two main conventions that we follow in the book are the same as in Van Oijen (2020):

1. Square brackets are used with probabilities, probability distributions, expectations and likelihoods: $p[\theta|y]$, $N[\mu, \sigma^2]$, $E[x]$, $L[\theta]$ etc.
2. Parentheses are used for functions, such as $f(x, \theta)$.

Outline of Chapters

We use the following abbreviations (which will be formally introduced in Chap. 1): x is the environmental variable of interest, z is the system response variable, $p[H]$ is the probability that the environmental variable is hazardous, V is the vulnerability of the system and R is the risk defined as expectation of loss.

This book consists of four parts. Chapters 1–11 focus on *probabilistic risk analysis* (PRA). Chapters 12–15 introduce *Bayesian decision theory* (BDT). Chapters 16–18 examine the link between PRA and BDT. Chapter 19 is a general discussion.

- **Chapter 1** begins with a short technical summary of the state of the art in PRA, identifying the key formulas and computer code. Then **three ways of classifying PRAs** are introduced. The first classification (Fig. 1.2) is according to the **number of components** into which risk is decomposed. The second classification (Fig. 1.3) is according to **resolution**, i.e. do we use one or more discrete classes of hazardous conditions H, or do we examine a continuum of possible hazard levels. The third classification (Fig. 1.4) is according to **implementation method**, i.e. do we use a distribution-based, sampling-based or model-based approach.
- **Chapter 2** derives the **basic formulas for distribution-based single-threshold PRA**, and shows under which conditions V would be constant. The formulas are applied to a Gaussian bivariate distribution $p[x, z]$ which implies a linear relationship. Specifically for this linear example, the chapter also derives formulas that allow a quick but approximate estimation of $p[H]$, V and R from basic properties of the distribution.
- **Chapter 3** shows equations and code for **sampling-based PRA**. The code is used to examine how sensitive the PRA is to the choice of hazard-threshold. This is done for the standard linear Gaussian example (of the preceding and other chapters) and for a nonlinear example.
- **Chapter 4** extends the sampling-based PRA with **uncertainty quantification**. It is tested on the same linear and nonlinear examples as before.
- **Chapter 5** is brief and shows how **density estimation** (fitting a distribution to a sample $\{(x_i, z_i)\}$) allows us to move from sampling-based to distribution-based PRA. It is explained using the linear example and results are compared to those of Chap. 3.
- **Chapter 6** introduces **copulas** as a flexible way of building a joint distribution for x and z from the marginal distributions. Code examples are provided that make use of the R-package `copula`. A wide range of joint probability distributions is presented.
- **Chapter 7** introduces a **Bayesian approach to model-based PRA**. Prior uncertainties for parameters and hyperparameters are specified, and Bayesian calibration is used to derive posterior probability distributions for use in PRA. Code examples use the R-package `Nimble`.
- **Chapter 8** shows how the equations for **multi-threshold PRA** (derived in Chapter 1) can be implemented in R-code, and results for the linear example are given.
- **Chapter 9** implements the equations for **continuous PRA** from Chap. 1 and applies them to the linear example.
- **Chapter 10** shows that the hazardous region can be subdivided in different ways than through a series of x-intervals (as in the multi-threshold PRA of Chap. 8), by distinguishing different **categories of hazard**. An example is given where the hazard is split up between stand-alone droughts and secondary droughts that follow an earlier drought in the immediately preceding time step. This is illustrated using a spatial example, where 64 PRAs are carried out in parallel on each of the cells in a 8×8 grid.

- **Chapter 11** discusses the consequences for the risk analysis of adding a third component to the risk decomposition, namely the degree of **exposure** of the ecosystem to the hazard. This is illustrated using the same spatial example as in the preceding chapter, with exposure being defined as the fraction of cells subject to drought.
- **Chapter 12** introduces **Bayesian decision theory** (BDT).
- **Chapter 13** shows how BDT can be represented with **graphical models** (Bayesian networks) and provides **analytical and numerical methods** for working with these models.
- **Chapter 14** analyses a **spatial example** in which decision makers have to decide where irrigation yields an increase in expected utility. The chapter also introduces model **emulation** as a stochastic but sometimes computationally efficient way of using deterministic models.
- **Chapter 15** carries out the BDT for the spatial example and shows that the use of emulation in risk analysis and decision-making comes with its own risks.
- **Chapter 16** studies the family relationships between PRA and BDT. It shows that minimisation of the risk to utility makes the methods equivalent.
- **Chapter 17 verifies the results** from the preceding chapter for the spatial example.
- **Chapter 18** is a very brief chapter, again on the spatial example, that shows **decomposition of risk into three components** rather than two.
- **Chapter 19** is a **general discussion** of the theory for PRA developed in this book, and its linkages to BDT.

Edinburgh, UK   Marcel van Oijen
Aberdeen, UK   Mark Brewer

Acknowledgements

This book is an outcome from the projects Carbo-extreme (funded by the European Union) and PRAFOR (funded by the United Kingdom's department for research and innovation, UKRI, within its Landscape Decisions programme). We thank the funders as well as our colleagues in the two projects. Danny Williamson (University of Exeter) and David Cameron (UK Centre for Ecology and Hydrology) provided helpful comments on the work. Marcel also wants to thank Eva Hiripi, his editor at Springer, for her enthusiasm and diligent work on this book and his earlier compendium of Bayesian methods.

Contents

Chapter 1
Introduction to Probabilistic Risk Analysis (PRA)

1.1 From Risk Matrices to PRA

In this book, we use the common definition of *risk* as the expectation of loss or damage due to some hazard (UN, 1992). *Risk analysis* seeks to decompose a risk into its constituent factors. This can be done by setting up a so-called *risk matrix*, and we show a typical example in Table 1.1. The matrix distinguishes different levels of two dimensions: (1) the probability of the hazard occurring, (2) the consequences of the hazard when it does occur. In our example, there are three levels to both dimensions, leading to nine possible combinations. If we assign numerical values to our two dimensions, we may quantify the risk as the product of the two values. This is shown in the nine cells of the matrix, with risks ranging from 1 to 9. Different risk values may motivate different actions.

Risk matrices are used often, for example in aviation and government (HM_Government, 2020). However, the approach is coarse, only semi-quantitative, and does not rigorously scale risk as the expectation of loss (Cox, 2008; Khan et al., 2020; Thomas et al., 2014). It is better to use a more formal form of quantitative risk analysis.

Whatever our system of interest is, we can only measure or estimate its variables with some degree of uncertainty. To account for these uncertainties, we will quantify all variables by means of probability distributions. Our approach to risk analysis thus will be an example of *probabilistic risk analysis* (PRA; Bedford & Cooke, 2001; Field et al., 2012). Our proposed methodology is inspired by ideas from the literature on PRA (first reviewed by Kaplan and Garrick (1981)), but we aim to make risk analysis more comprehensively probabilistic.

Previous implementations of PRA have tended to focus on risks associated with discrete hazardous events (earthquakes, nuclear meltdowns, epidemics, etc.) and discrete states of system "failure," but we want our approach to be generally applicable. Therefore, risk decomposition as we define it in our PRA framework

M. van Oijen, M. Brewer, *Probabilistic Risk Analysis and Bayesian Decision Theory*, SpringerBriefs in Statistics, https://doi.org/10.1007/978-3-031-16333-3_1

Table 1.1 Typical risk matrix

Consequence	Probability	1 (unlikely)	2 (medium)	3 (likely)
1 (minor)		1	2	3
2 (medium)		2	4	6
3 (major)		3	6	9

is not equivalent to "fault tree analysis" (FTA) in engineering projects (Rausand, 2020). FTA quantifies the probability of failure for the key components in a human-made system and this is modelled using discrete probability distributions. This approach is not suitable for application in disciplines like ecology and environmental science where response variables tend to be continuous rather than binary. Crop growth or biodiversity do not abruptly "fail" when there is a drought or pollution, instead they can change to any given degree. Therefore our framework for risk analysis will make use of continuous probability distributions and define vulnerability as a function of expectation values and not discrete probabilities. We have not found the PRA equations that we will propose here (beginning in the next section of this chapter) in the engineering literature, although of course there is conceptual similarity between risk analyses in different fields.

1.2 Basic Equations for PRA

Our development of PRA starts by defining risk as the statistical expectation of loss. We will show that this expectation can be decomposed formally following the rules of probability theory, without the use of risk matrices.

PRA, as developed in recent publications (Van Oijen et al., 2014, 2013; Van Oijen & Zavala, 2019), studies the relationship between an environmental variable (x) and a system variable (z) (Fig. 1.1). The PRA-method can be applied to any set of (x, z)-values, irrespective of the nature of their relationship. The method allows for the response of z to x to change over time, which should show up in the analysis as a change in *vulnerability* of the system. The results from the PRA depend on a subjective choice for how we divide the x-domain into *hazardous* and *non-hazardous* regions, denoted as H and $\neg H$. Usually this means setting a threshold below or above which x is considered hazardous.

One nice aspect of this way of working (which only uses model I-O or observations of (x, z), and does not require examining the underlying modelled or real mechanisms nor carries out any regression of z on x) is that the method is fast. Once the threshold has been set, it is a very simple calculation to calculate the hazard probability $p[H]$, the vulnerability V and the risk R.

As mentioned, our PRA uses the standard definition for risk (R) as being the expectation of loss. More concretely, R is the difference between what the system could achieve on average if hazardous conditions (H) never occurred, and what it

Fig. 1.1 PRA as a
probabilistic network

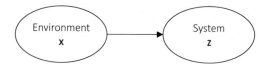

actually does achieve. We can write this as the expectation for the z-variable under non-hazardous conditions minus its overall expectation for any conditions:

$$R = E[z|\neg H] - E[z], \tag{1.1}$$

where $\neg H$ stands for non-hazardous environmental conditions. The probability of hazardous environmental conditions is denoted as $p[H]$, so the probability of non-hazardous conditions is $1 - p[H]$. Vulnerability V is implicitly defined by requiring that $R = p[H] \times V$, so that:

$$
\begin{aligned}
V &= R \,/\, p[H] \\
&= (E[z|\neg H] - E[z]) \,/\, p[H] \\
&= (E[z|\neg H] - p[H]E[z|H] - (1 - p[H])E[z|\neg H]) \,/\, p[H] \\
&= E[z|\neg H] - E[z|H].
\end{aligned}
\tag{1.2}
$$

This definition of V is the only possible one if R is defined as expected loss and also as the product of $p[H]$ and V. It stands in contrast to the many different definitions of vulnerability that can be found in the literature on environmental risk analysis, most of which cannot be put in a consistent mathematical framework.

So here is our basic approach to PRA in a nutshell:

1. R is expected loss,
2. V is expectation for non-hazardous conditions minus that for hazardous conditions,
3. R can be decomposed as the product of $p[H]$ and V.

We shall refine this approach in various ways, but always aim to maintain mathematical consistency between the various components of risk.

1.3   Decomposition of Risk: 2 or 3 Components

The main strength of our approach to PRA is that it allows formal decomposition of risk into different components (Fig. 1.2). In our introduction above we indicated how risk can be decomposed into two components: $R = p[H] \times V$, and that is the decomposition that we shall be using the most in this book. However, it is possible to add a third component, *exposure* Q, so that we can write: $R = p[H] \times Q \times V$,

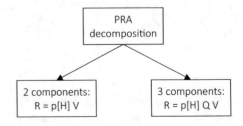

Fig. 1.2 PRA-classification according to treatment of the hazardous region

without changing the definition of V but with consequences for how we interpret R. Such decomposition into three components will be discussed briefly in Chap. 11.

1.4 Resolution of PRA: Single-Threshold, Multi-Threshold, Categorical, Continuous

The above definitions apply irrespective of whether z and x are discrete or continuous variables. But our applications will mostly be for variables that are continuous. For example, z could be the growth of a forest and x could be the amount of available water. In such cases hazardous conditions will generally be defined using intervals of x-values. Hazardous conditions could arise when a given x-variable moves below or above a threshold, or exceeds a central interval in either direction. The x-variable could even be multivariate, in which case the hazardous region is not an interval but a region, possibly disjoint, in a higher-dimensional space.

For ease of exposition, and without loss of generality, we shall in this book only discuss cases where x is a continuous scalar variable and hazards are low values of x. In most cases, threshold-values of x will be used to define hazardous regions. We can distinguish different types of PRA depending on the number of thresholds that are specified (Fig. 1.3):

Fig. 1.3 PRA-classification according to treatment of the hazardous region

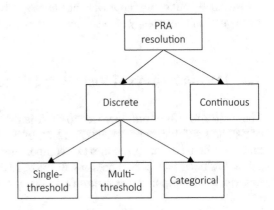

- PRA that uses only one threshold-value to define a single hazardous region H.
- PRA that uses a series of thresholds to define multiple hazardous regions $\{H_i\}$, $i = 1..n$.
- PRA where the number of thresholds goes to infinity and the sizes of $\{H_i\}$ go to zero.

Additionally, we distinguish a fourth type:

- PRA that defines multiple hazardous regions $\{H_i\}$ not through a threshold-series but by recognizing different *categories* of hazard.

We refer to the 'infinite thresholds' PRA as *continuous PRA* and to the others as *discrete PRA*. Let's now consider all four types of PRA in turn.

1.4.1 Single-Threshold PRA

In *single-threshold PRA*, hazardous conditions are those where the x-variable has dropped below a given threshold. In that case, $E[z|H] = E[z|x < thr]$ and $E[z|\neg H] = E[z|x \geq thr]$. So our PRA-equations become:

$$
\begin{aligned}
V &= E[z|x \geq thr] - E[z|x < thr], \\
R &= E[z|x \geq thr] - E[z] \\
  &= p[H]\,V.
\end{aligned}
\tag{1.3}
$$

- Many examples of PRA in this book will be single-threshold PRA, but more complex PRAs will be presented as well.

1.4.2 Multi-Threshold PRA

In *multi-threshold PRA*, we define $n \geq 2$ thresholds, with thr_1 being the smallest and thr_n the largest. This divides the hazardous region into n different intervals. We then carry out a separate PRA for each interval using the following equations:

$$
\begin{aligned}
p[H_i] &= p[thr_{i-1} \leq x < thr_i], \\
V_i &= E[z|\neg H] - E[z|H_i] \\
    &= E[z|x \geq thr_n] - E[z|thr_{i-1} \leq x < thr_i], \\
R_i &= p[H_i]\,V_i,
\end{aligned}
\tag{1.4}
$$

for $i = 1, .., n$ and where $thr_0 = -\infty$. Note that these equations for multi-threshold PRA simplify to Eq. (1.3) when $n = 1$. But even when $n \geq 2$ we can retrieve the single-threshold PRA for the whole hazardous region by summing the results for the different intervals:

$$p[H] = \sum p[H_i],$$

$$V = \sum \frac{p[H_i]}{p[H]} V_i,$$

$$R = \sum R_i,$$

$$= p[H] V, \tag{1.5}$$

with all summations running from $i = 1$ to n.

Multi-threshold PRA thus is a refinement of single-threshold PRA if they share the same non-hazardous region, i.e. if the highest threshold thr_n of the former is chosen to be the same as the single threshold thr of the latter. In that case Eq. (1.5) returns the same overall values for $p[H]$, V and R as Eq. (1.3) does. But multi-threshold PRA then gives us additional information about the relative probabilities and vulnerabilities for the n different sub-levels of the hazardous region.

- We show an example of multi-threshold PRA in action in Chap. 8.

1.4.3 Categorical PRA

In *categorical PRA*, we assume that the hazardous region is the union of multiple categories of hazard. This can be done in many different ways, but in all cases the approach and the equations are very similar to those of multi-threshold PRA. The only difference is that the various H_i are not defined by a series of x-thresholds but by some other distinguishing criteria.

- We show an example of categorical PRA in Chap. 10.

1.4.4 Continuous PRA

In multi-threshold discrete PRA we can specify as many hazard levels as we want. In the limit of $n \to \infty$ we arrive at a continuous formulation of PRA which only keeps the single highest threshold-level ($thr = thr_n$):

$$R = \int_{x=-\infty}^{thr} r(x)dx, \tag{1.6}$$

where

$$r(x) = p[x] \, v(x),$$
$$v(x) = E[z|x \geq thr] - E[z|x].$$

(1.7)

We can take this one step further and remove the need to specify a threshold altogether if we replace $E[z|x \geq thr]$ with a constant $\max_{x \in X} E[z|x]$.

• We show an application of continuous PRA in Chap. 9.

1.5   Implementation of PRA: Distribution-Based, Sampling-Based, Model-Based

If the joint distribution $p[x, z]$ is available to us in closed form, we can write down equations for the conditional expectations that we need in PRA. But if not, we may estimate the expectations from a sample of observations $\{(x_i, z_i)\}$. We refer to these two methods as *distribution-based* and *sampling-based* PRA, respectively (Fig. 1.4). Of course, when all we have is a sample, we could fit a joint distribution to the data and then proceed with distribution-based PRA. A third method involves fitting not a distribution but a statistical model, e.g. a regression model, and we refer to this as *model-based* PRA (Fig. 1.4). If the model is fit by means of Bayesian calibration, the PRA can be carried out on the posterior probability distribution for all uncertain quantities.

• Examples of distribution-based PRA can be found in Chaps. 2, 5, 6 and 9.
• Examples of sampling-based PRA can be found in Chaps. 3, 4, 8, 10 and 11.
• Examples of model-based PRA can be found in Chap. 7.

Fig. 1.4 PRA-classification according to implementation method

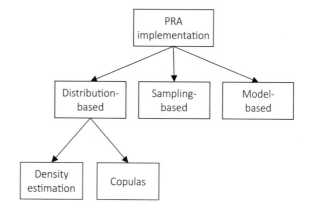

Chapter 2
Distribution-Based Single-Threshold PRA

2.1 Conditional Distributions for z

Equation (1.3) shows that the key probability distributions for basic PRA are $p[z|x < thr]$ and $p[z|x \geq thr]$. These are derived as the ratio of joint and marginal distributions:

$$
\begin{aligned}
p[z|x < thr] &= \frac{p[z, x < thr]}{p[x < thr]} \\
&= \frac{p[z] \int_{x=-\infty}^{thr} p[x|z]\, dx}{p[x < thr]} \\
&= \frac{p[z] F_{x|z}[thr]}{F_x[thr]}, \\
p[z|x \geq thr] &= \frac{p[z](1 - F_{x|z}[thr])}{1 - F_x[thr]},
\end{aligned}
\tag{2.1}
$$

where $F_x[thr]$ and $F_{x|z}[thr]$ are the cumulative distribution functions associated with $p[x]$ and $p[x|z]$, both evaluated at $x = thr$. Note that $F_x[thr] = p[x < thr]$ is the hazard probability $p[H]$.

Supplementary Information The online version contains supplementary material available at https://doi.org/10.1007/978-3-031-16333-3_2

From our formulas for the conditional distributions (Eq. (2.1)), we can derive the two conditional expectations that we need for the single-threshold PRA (Eq. (1.3)):

$$E[z|x < thr] = \int_{z=-\infty}^{\infty} z\, p[z|x < thr]\, dz$$

$$= \frac{1}{F_x[thr]} \int_{z=-\infty}^{\infty} z\, p[z]\, F_{x|z}[thr]\, dz, \qquad (2.2)$$

$$E[z|x \geq thr] = \frac{1}{1 - F_x[thr]} \int_{z=-\infty}^{\infty} z\, p[z]\, (1 - F_{x|z}[thr])\, dz.$$

These conditional expectations involve integrals over z, but we can also use integrals over x:

$$E[z|x < thr] = \frac{1}{F_x[thr]} \int_{x=-\infty}^{thr} p[x]\, E[z|x]\, dx,$$

$$\qquad (2.3)$$

$$E[z|x \geq thr] = \frac{1}{1 - F_x[thr]} \int_{x=thr}^{\infty} p[x]\, E[z|x]\, dx.$$

2.1.1 Conditions for V Being Constant

From the last equation we can derive how vulnerability V changes with the value of the threshold thr:

$$\frac{d V}{d\, thr} = \frac{d\, (E[z|x \geq thr] - E[z|x < thr])}{d\, thr}$$

$$= p[thr]\{ \frac{E[z|x \geq thr] - z[thr]}{1 - F_x[thr]} - \frac{z[thr] - E[z|x < thr]}{F_x[thr]} \} \qquad (2.4)$$

$$= \frac{p[thr]}{F_x[thr](1 - F_x[thr])} \{E[z|x \geq thr]F_x[thr] - z[thr]$$

$$+ E[z|x < thr](1 - F_x[thr])\},$$

where $z[thr] = E[z|x = thr]$. So V is locally constant at $x = thr$ when the term between curly brackets is zero. Let's use Eq. (2.4) to find a combination of hazard distribution $p[x]$ and response function $z[x]$ for which vulnerability is constant. Consider a linear response $z[x] = a + b\,x$ with a uniformly distributed environmental variable $x \sim U[0, 1]$. Then $p[thr] = 1$, $F_x[thr] = thr$, $E[z|x < thr] = a + b\,thr/2$, $E[z \geq thr] = a + b(thr + 1)/2$ and we find, after substitution in Eq. (2.4), that V is constant over the whole range of x.

2.2 Example of Distribution-Based PRA: Gaussian $p[x, z]$

Equations (2.2) and (2.3) show two ways in which we can implement the single-threshold PRA for any joint probability distribution for (x, z). The next section shows an example where $p[x, z]$ is a bivariate Gaussian probability distribution. After that, we shall discuss the PRA for the more common situation where we do not have an explicit joint distribution $p[x, z]$ but just a sample of joint observations $\{(x_i, z_i), i = 1..n\}$.

Say that our joint probability distribution for x and z is the following:

EXAMPLE: Bivariate Gaussian for x and z:

$p[x, z] = N[\mu, \Sigma]$, where

$$\mu = \begin{bmatrix} \mu_x \\ \mu_z \end{bmatrix} = \begin{bmatrix} 0 \\ 0 \end{bmatrix}; \quad \Sigma = \begin{bmatrix} \sigma_x^2 & \rho \sigma_x \sigma_z \\ \rho \sigma_x \sigma_z & \sigma_z^2 \end{bmatrix} = \begin{bmatrix} 1 & 0.5 \\ 0.5 & 1 \end{bmatrix}.$$

(2.5)

The marginal and conditional distributions are then:

$$p[x] = N[\mu_x, \sigma_x^2] = N[0, 1],$$

$$p[z] = N[\mu_z, \sigma_z^2] = N[0, 1],$$

$$p[z|x] = N[\mu_z + \rho(x - \mu_x)\frac{\sigma_z}{\sigma_x}, \sigma_z^2(1 - \rho^2)] = N[0.5x, 0.75].$$

(2.6)

We show $p[x]$, $p[z]$, $p[x, z]$, and three examples of $p[z|x]$ in Fig. 2.1.

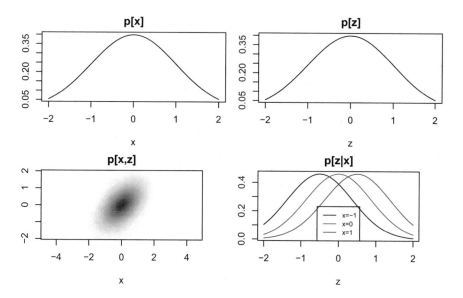

Fig. 2.1 Marginal, joint, and conditional Gaussian distributions for x and z

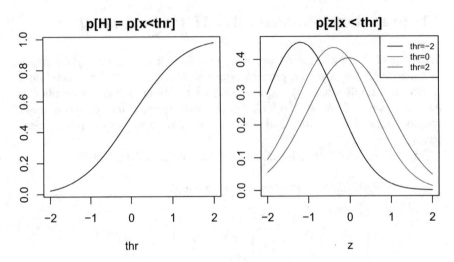

Fig. 2.2 $p[H]$ and $p[z|x < thr]$ for the bivariate Gaussian

2.2.1   Hazard Probability and Conditional Distributions

The hazard probability $p[H] = p[x < thr]$ is equal to the cumulative distribution function evaluated at $x = thr$, and we denote this as $F_x[thr]$. We show $p[H]$ as a function of the threshold-value in the left panel of Fig. 2.2.

The right panel of Fig. 2.2 shows, for three values of the threshold, the conditional probability distribution $p[z|H] = p[z|x < thr]$.

2.2.2   Conditional Expectations and PRA

We are now ready to calculate and plot the conditional expectations that we need for our PRA according to Eq. (1.3) and for which we derived the integrals of Eqs. (2.2) and (2.3). We choose to implement the latter equation. However, the integrals in that equation cannot be analytically solved, so we discretize the domain of x and approximate the integrals with sums. Our discretization uses 101 values of x uniformly spaced between 0 and 5 standard deviations from the threshold. Here is our R-code that calculates the first integral (the code for the second is similar) for any choice of threshold-value thr:

```
Ez_xbelow <- function(thr=0, mz.=mz, mx.=mx, Vz.=Vz, Vx.=Vx, r=rxz) {
    x.seq    <- seq( thr-5*sqrt(Vx.), thr, length.out=101 )
    px.seq   <- px( x.seq, m=mx., V=Vx. ) ; px.sum <- sum(px.seq)
    Ez_x.seq <- mz. + r * (x.seq-mx.) * sqrt(Vz./Vx.)
    Ezxbelow <- sum(px.seq * Ez_x.seq) / px.sum
    return( Ezxbelow ) }
```

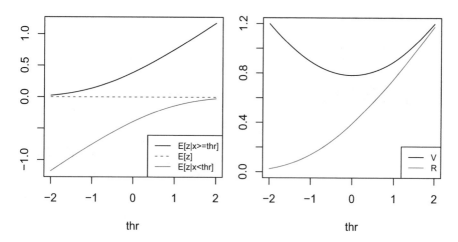

Fig. 2.3 Distribution-based single-threshold PRA: bivariate Gaussian example. Left: conditional expectations for z as a function of threshold-value. Right: the corresponding values of V and R

We use these R-functions to calculate the expectations for a range of threshold-values, as shown in the left panel of Fig. 2.3. That completes the preparation for this distribution-based single-threshold PRA and the values of V and R for the whole range of threshold-values are shown in the right panel of the same figure.

2.3 Approximation Formulas for the Conditional Bivariate Gaussian Expectations

Even though in the case of the bivariate Gaussian no closed-form solution exists for the distribution of z given that x is below or above a threshold, there is an approximation formula for $E[z|x < thr]$ that works quite well. Mee and Owen (1983) provide this for the standard bivariate Gaussian as $E[z|x < thr] \approx -\rho\, p_x[thr]/F_x[thr]$. Let's generalise this formula to any bivariate normal and to $E[z|x \geq thr]$:

APPRXOXIMATION FOR BIVARIATE GAUSSIAN p[x,z]:

$$E[z|x < thr] \approx E[z] - \rho\, \sigma_x\, \sigma_z\, \frac{p_x[thr]}{F_x[thr]},$$

$$E[z|x \geq thr] \approx E[z] + \rho\, \sigma_x\, \sigma_z\, \frac{p_x[thr]}{1 - F_x[thr]}.$$

(2.7)

Fig. 2.4 Conditional
expectations for z as a
function of threshold-value in
the case of bivariate Gaussian
$p[x, z]$. Solid lines: Monte
Carlo sampling (MC). Dashed
lines: approximation formulas

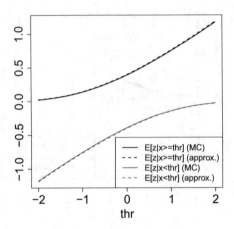

We implement these formulas in R and in Fig. 2.4 compare their performance
with the Monte Carlo estimates that we found before in the left panel of Fig. 2.3.
The results are near-identical so the approximation is very good.

Note that Eq. (2.7) allows for a very simple approximate PRA for the bivariate
Gaussian:

APPROXIMATE PRA FOR BIVARIATE GAUSSIAN p[x,z]:

$$p[H] = F_x[thr],$$

$$V \approx \frac{\rho \, \sigma_x \, \sigma_z \, p_x[thr]}{F_x[thr] \, (1 - F_x[thr])},$$ (2.8)

$$R \approx \frac{\rho \, \sigma_x \, \sigma_z \, p_x[thr]}{1 - F_x[thr]}.$$

Chapter 3
Sampling-Based Single-Threshold PRA

In applications, we do not have a pre-specified joint distribution for x and z, but we have a sample of observations as in the left panel of Fig. 3.1. So we cannot use the functions defined above for the distribution-based PRA. Instead, we must estimate the PRA-integrals by sampling. The probabilities $p[.]$ are then replaced by normalised frequencies, but we shall denote those with $p[.]$ too. Say the total number of (x, z) observations is n of which n_H have x-values that are below a threshold thr. We then write, as before, $p[x < thr] = p[H]$ and estimate this as n_H/n. We denote the set of z-values in the interval $x < thr$ as $z_H = \{z_H(i); i = 1..n_H\}$, and the complement as $z_{\neg H}$. We then estimate the three expectations needed for the PRA as:

<u>SAMPLE MEANS:</u>

$$
\begin{aligned}
\hat{E}[z] &= \bar{z}, \\
\hat{E}[z|x < thr] &= \overline{z_H}, \\
\hat{E}[z|x \geq thr] &= \overline{z_{\neg H}}.
\end{aligned}
\tag{3.1}
$$

The sampling-based PRA uses these estimates of expectations to estimate V and R, instead of the distribution-based values given in Eqs. (2.2) and (2.3). The sample

---

Supplementary Information The online version contains supplementary material available at https://doi.org/10.1007/978-3-031-16333-3_3

M. van Oijen, M. Brewer, *Probabilistic Risk Analysis and Bayesian Decision Theory*, SpringerBriefs in Statistics, https://doi.org/10.1007/978-3-031-16333-3_3

means are unbiased estimators of the true means. We implement the sample-based
PRA as follows in R:

```
PRA <- function( x, z, thr=0 ) {
  n  <- length(z) ; H    <- which(x < thr) ; nH      <- length(H)
  Ez <- mean( z ) ; Ez_H <- mean( z[H] )   ; Ez_notH <- mean( z[-H] )
  pH <- nH / n    ; V     <- Ez_notH - Ez_H ; R       <- Ez_notH - Ez
  return( c(pH=pH,V=V,R=R) ) }
```

3.1 Example of Sampling-Based PRA: Linear Relationship

We apply the PRA-code to the sample data set shown on the left in Fig. 3.1, which
was generated from the same bivariate Gaussian distribution that we used above.
We choose a threshold-value: $thr = 0$. The values for V and R estimated from the
sample are shown on the right.

3.1.1 Varying the Threshold

Using the same data set, we vary the threshold value from -2 to 2, and show what
that means for the estimates of $p[H]$, V and R in Fig. 3.2. As we would expect, the
results are not smooth because of sampling variation. But overall the estimates show
the same dependency on the threshold-value that we found before when we worked
directly with the bivariate Gaussian rather than a finite sample from it (Fig. 2.2 left
panel, Fig. 2.3 right panel).

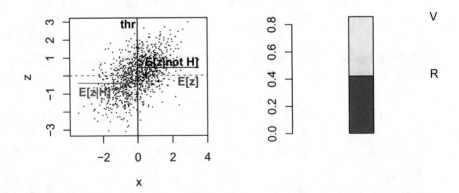

Fig. 3.1 Sampling-based single-threshold PRA on 'data set 1' with thr = 0. Left: data and
expectation values. Right: V and R

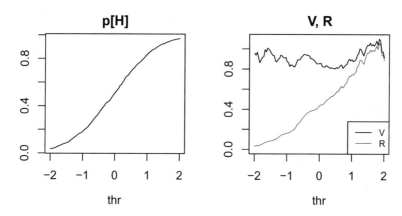

Fig. 3.2 Sampling-based single-threshold PRA on data set 1 for a range of different thresholds. Left: $p[H]$. Right: V and R

3.2 Example of Sampling-Based PRA: Nonlinear Relationship

The sampling-based procedure can be applied irrespective of how x and z are related. To show this, we now take a sample from the following noisy nonlinear relationship:

NONLINEAR RELATIONSHIP BETWEEN x AND z:

$$z|x \sim N[f(x), \sigma_z^2], \quad x \geq 0, where \tag{3.2}$$

$$f(x) = 1 - exp(-x).$$

So we have $E[z|x] = f(x) = 1 - exp(-x)$. Let's further assume that x is uniformly distributed in the interval [0,3] and that $\sigma_z^2 = 0.01$. We take a sample from $p[x, z] = p[x]p[z|x]$ and apply the PRA: see Fig. 3.3. The results are not dramatically different from those for the linear (bivariate Gaussian) relationship between x and z. The only difference is that V decreases continuously with the value of the threshold thr. This is because the relationship between x and z is concave and therefore the benefit to z of x being above the threshold decreases with thr.

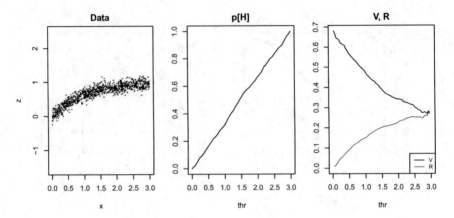

Fig. 3.3 PRA on a data set from a nonlinear relationship

Chapter 4
Sampling-Based Single-Threshold PRA: Uncertainty Quantification (UQ)

Uncertainty in sampling-based expectations may be quantified as the standard deviations of the sample means, see Eq. (4.1):

STANDARD DEVIATIONS OF SAMPLE MEANS:

$$
\begin{aligned}
\sigma_{\hat{E}[z]} &= \sqrt{\frac{Var[z]}{n}}, \\[2mm]
\sigma_{\hat{E}[z|x<thr]} &= \sqrt{\frac{Var[z_H]}{n_H}}, \\[2mm]
\sigma_{\hat{E}[z|x\geq thr]} &= \sqrt{\frac{Var[z_{\neg H}]}{n - n_H}}.
\end{aligned}
\tag{4.1}
$$

Uncertainties for vulnerability (V) and risk (R), both of which are defined as differences of expectations, can be calculated as the square root of the sum of the two relevant σ^2-values, corrected for the covariance (in the case of R). Before implementing these uncertainty calculations in R, we note two caveats:

- Variances of sample means are estimated without bias (as the sample variance divided by n), but taking the square root is a nonlinear operation so the standard deviation estimates are biased (in fact underestimates because of Jensen's inequality and the fact that $\sqrt{()}$ is a strictly concave function). This will not be a major problem if n is high enough.
- Standard deviations do not imply unique credibility intervals, unless we can assume that the underlying distributions are Gaussian. However, Chebyshev's

Supplementary Information The online version contains supplementary material available at https://doi.org/10.1007/978-3-031-16333-3_4

M. van Oijen, M. Brewer, *Probabilistic Risk Analysis and Bayesian Decision Theory*, SpringerBriefs in Statistics, https://doi.org/10.1007/978-3-031-16333-3_4

inequality (which states that at most $1/k^2$ of probability mass is outside k standard deviations from the mean) may be used to calculate conservative uncertainty intervals. For example, the *mean* $\pm\, 2\sigma$ would constitute an 'at least 75% probability interval.'

We now turn to the calculation of uncertainties in $p[H]$, V and R.

4.1   Uncertainty in $p[H]$

We represent our uncertainty about the occurrence of hazardous conditions as a binomial distribution with proportion parameter $p[H]$. This choice implies that we believe that hazardous conditions appear independently: given a value for $p[H]$, knowledge of a hazard in the recent past or a nearby location does not provide any information about the hazard probability here and now.

As indicated above, we estimate $p[H]$ as the relative frequency of hazard occurrences in our x-data. That implies that we started from a uniform prior $U[0, 1]$ for $p[H]$, which is the same as a $Be[1, 1]$ beta-distribution. The beta-binomial combination is conjugate, so the posterior uncertainty can be found analytically (Van Oijen, 2020, Chap. 5) as follows:

<u>POSTERIOR UNCERTAINTY FOR $p[H]$</u> :

$$p[H] \sim Be[a, b] \implies$$

$$\sigma_{p[H]} = \frac{1}{a+b}\sqrt{\frac{ab}{a+b+1}},$$

(4.2)

where $a = 1 + n_H$ and $b = 1 + n - n_H$.

4.2   Uncertainty in V

We continue with the sampling-based single-threshold PRA. Vulnerability is defined as $V = E[z \geq thr] - E[z < thr]$, which we estimate from the observations as the difference between $\overline{z_{\neg H}}$ and $\overline{z_H}$. The two terms refer to non-overlapping subsets of the observations z, so the variances for the two terms can be added which gives us the following uncertainty for the estimate of V:

<u>POSTERIOR UNCERTAINTY FOR V</u> :

$$\sigma_V = \sqrt{\sigma^2_{\hat{E}[z|x \geq thr]} + \sigma^2_{\hat{E}[z|x < thr]}},$$

(4.3)

where $\sigma_{\hat{E}[z|x \geq thr]}$ and $\sigma_{\hat{E}[z|x < thr]}$ are as defined in Eq. (4.1).

4.3   Uncertainty in R

In this section we derive an equation for σ_R which improves on the one provided by Van Oijen and Zavala (2019).

Risk is defined as $R = E[z \geq thr] - E[z]$, which we estimate from the observations as the difference between $\overline{z_{\neg H}}$ and $\overline{z}$. In contrast to V, these two terms represent overlapping (sub)sets of the observations z, so the sum of variances for the two terms must be corrected for covariance (because $Var[A - B] = Var[A] + Var[B] - 2\,Cov[A, B]$, where $Cov[A, B] = E[(A - \overline{A})(B - \overline{B})]$). Here the overlapping region is $\neg H$ which contains a fraction $1 - n_H/n$ of the observations. So any deviation $\overline{z_{\neg H}} - E[z \geq thr]$ is expected to coincide with a deviation $\overline{z} - E[z]$ that is a fraction n_H/n smaller. So the covariance is $(1 - \frac{n_H}{n})\sigma^2_{\hat{E}[z|x\geq thr]}$ which gives the following equation for uncertainty about a sample-based estimate for R:

POSTERIOR UNCERTAINTY FOR R :

$$\sigma_R = \sqrt{\sigma^2_{\hat{E}[z|x\geq thr]} + \sigma^2_{\hat{E}[z]} - 2(1 - \frac{n_H}{n})\sigma^2_{\hat{E}[z|x\geq thr]}}, \qquad (4.4)$$

where $\sigma_{\hat{E}[z|x\geq thr]}$ and $\sigma_{\hat{E}[z]}$ are as defined in Eq. (4.1).

4.4   Extension of R-Code for PRA: Adding the UQ

We now add the above equations for UQ to the R-function for PRA that we showed before:

```
PRA.UQ <- function( x, z, thr=0 ) {
  n  <- length(z) ; H    <- which(x < thr) ; nH       <- length(H)
  Ez <- mean( z ) ; Ez_H <- mean( z[H] )   ; Ez_notH <- mean( z[-H] )
  pH <- nH / n    ; V    <- Ez_notH - Ez_H ; R        <- Ez_notH - Ez

  a          <- 1 + nH ; b    <- 1 + n - nH
  s_Ez       <- sqrt( var(z    ) / n     )
  s_Ez_H     <- sqrt( var(z[ H]) /   nH  )
  s_Ez_notH  <- sqrt( var(z[-H]) / (n-nH) )

  s_pH <- sqrt( a*b/(a+b+1) ) / (a+b)
  s_V  <- sqrt( s_Ez_notH^2 + s_Ez_H^2 )
  s_R  <- sqrt( s_Ez_notH^2 + s_Ez^2 - 2 * s_Ez_notH^2 * (1-nH/n) )

  return( c(pH=pH,V=V,R=R,s_pH=s_pH,s_V=s_V,s_R=s_R) )
}
```

4.5   PRA with UQ on the Nonlinear Data Set

We now repeat the last PRA of the preceding chapter, the one on the nonlinear data set (Fig. 3.3), this time adding the UQ. The new results are shown in the top panels of Fig. 4.1.

The bottom two panels of Fig. 4.1 show results for a random subsample of 10% from the same data. Because that sample is much smaller, all uncertainties are increased.

4.6   Verification of the UQ by Simulating Multiple Data Sets

In practice, we will be applying PRA with UQ to individual real data sets, and we can then use the above formulas for uncertainty estimation. But we can test whether the formulas are correct by simulating many data sets from an assumed joint distribution, and looking at the spread of the estimated values for $p[H]$, V and R. The spread of these values between simulated data sets should be about the same as indicated by our estimates for $\sigma_{p[H]}$, σ_V and σ_R derived from any single data set. This is what we now test for a joint probability distribution $p[x, z]$ that represents a noisy nonlinear (negative exponential) relationship between the two variables. That will be followed by a test where we use multiple samples from a linear relationship.

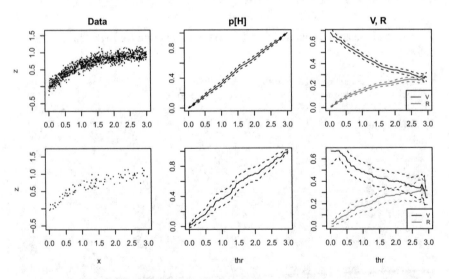

Fig. 4.1 PRA on nonlinearly related x and z, with UQ. Top row: as previous example. Bottom row: same but just 10% of data being used. Dashed lines are 2 standard deviations away from the mean

4.6.1   UQ-Verification: Nonlinear Relationship

We begin by generating $nd = 1000$ different data sets from $p[x, z]$, with each individual data set containing $n = 1000$ observations:

```
nd <- 1e3 ; listxz <- vector("list",nd) ; n  <- 1e3 ; sz <- 0.1
for(d in 1:nd) {
  x <- runif( n, 0, 3 ) ; ez <- rnorm( n, 0, sz) ; z <- 1-exp(-x) + ez
  listxz[[d]] <- cbind(x,z) }
```

The first three of the generated data sets are shown in Fig. 4.2.

Using the R-function that we defined above, we now carry out the PRA with UQ for each of the 1000 data sets, for a threshold value of $thr=1$, and store the results in a table:

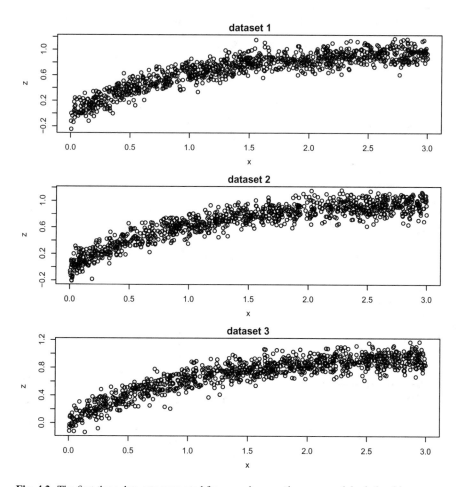

Fig. 4.2 The first three data sets generated from a noisy negative exponential relationship

```
thr      <- 1
PRA.tbl <- t( sapply( 1:nd, function(d){
  PRA.UQ( listxz[[d]][,"x"], listxz[[d]][,"z"], thr) } ) )
```

The first three rows of the table, i.e. the PRAs for the three sample data sets shown in Fig. 4.2, are as follows:

```
>           pH          V          R        s_pH        s_V          s_R
> [1,] 0.320 0.4732057 0.1514258 0.01473357 0.01298911 0.008124927
> [2,] 0.344 0.5008567 0.1722947 0.01500286 0.01328335 0.008803770
> [3,] 0.311 0.4681190 0.1455850 0.01462122 0.01250033 0.007879280
```

In that table, the uncertainty-estimates in the three rightmost columns are specific for the individual data sets, so each data set leads to slightly different uncertainty values. Better estimates of the uncertainties are produced by considering the spread of p[H], V and R between all 1000 data sets, for which we use the following R-code:

```
slist_pH <- sd( PRA.tbl[,"pH"] )
slist_V  <- sd( PRA.tbl[,"V" ] )
slist_R  <- sd( PRA.tbl[,"R" ] )
```

Figure 4.3 shows the results from carrying out 1000 different PRAs, each on a different realisation from the same 'nonlinear' joint distribution for x and z. Each

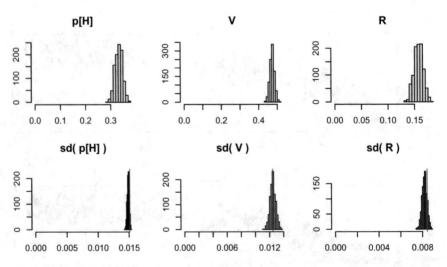

Fig. 4.3 PRAs on 1000 realisations (virtual data sets) from the same nonlinear relationship between x and z. Top row: distributions of the 1000 estimates for $p[H]$, V and R. Bottom row: distributions of the 1000 uncertainty estimates (sigma-values). The vertical red lines indicate the standard deviations of the top-row estimates (widths of top-row histograms)

realisation consisted of 1000 (x, z) pairs. From the figure, we can draw the following conclusions:

- The variation between the 1000 estimates for $p[H]$, V and R was fairly small. This was because each of the 1000 estimates was based on a large sample from $p[x, z]$.
- Likewise, the 1000 estimates of uncertainty $\sigma_{p[H]}$, σ_V and σ_R showed only minor variation.
- The 1000 realisation-specific estimates of $\sigma_{p[H]}$, σ_V and σ_R clustered closely around the standard deviations of the 1000 estimates of $p[H]$, V and R. This suggests that the uncertainties for all three risk analysis terms are well estimated from a sample of (x, z) using Eqs. (4.2), (4.3) and (4.4).

4.6.2   UQ-Verification: Linear Relationship

Above, we tested our UQ-equations for a nonlinear relationship between x and z. We now test the equations on 1000 different data sets from a bivariate Gaussian $p[x, z]$, i.e. a linear relationship:

```
mx   <- mz <- 0 ; Vx   <- Vz <- 1 ; rxz <- 0.5
mxz <- c(mx,mz)
Sxz <- diag( c(Vx,Vz) ) ; Sxz[1,2] <- Sxz[2,1] <- rxz * sqrt(Vx * Vz)

nd <- 1e3 ; listxz <- vector("list",nd) ; n  <- 1e3
for(d in 1:nd) {
  xz <- rmvnorm( n, mxz, Sxz ) ; x <- xz[,1] ; z <- xz[,2]
  listxz[[d]] <- cbind(x,z) }
```

The first three of the generated linear data sets are shown in Fig. 4.4.

We now carry out a PRA with UQ for each of the 1000 linear data sets, for a threshold value of $thr = -1$. The first three PRAs, for the three sample data sets shown in Fig. 4.4, are as follows:

```
>         pH         V         R       s_pH        s_V        s_R
> [1,] 0.157 1.0020492 0.1573217 0.01150752 0.07853827 0.01685975
> [2,] 0.172 0.9314785 0.1602143 0.01193389 0.07335956 0.01679685
> [3,] 0.143 0.9003982 0.1287569 0.01107661 0.08166846 0.01533052
```

As in the preceding section, the uncertainty-estimates on the right are specific to the individual data sets. And again, better global estimates of the uncertainties are produced by considering the spread of p[H], V and R between all 1000 data sets. We compare the two approaches in Fig. 4.5 and contrast the results for these linear data with our earlier findings for nonlinear data (Fig. 4.3):

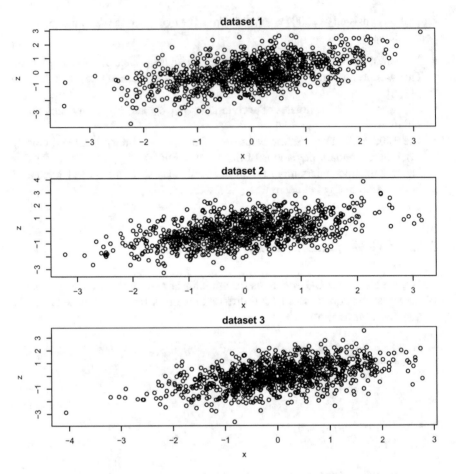

Fig. 4.4 The first three data sets generated from a noisy linear relationship

- We again see, in the bottom row of Fig. 4.5, that the 1000 uncertainty-estimates for $p[H]$, V and R all cluster around the correct values. This supports the value of Eqs. (4.1)–(4.4) for UQ of sampling-based PRA-terms.

4.7 Approximation Formulas for the Conditional Bivariate Gaussian Variances

Earlier we presented, for the bivariate Gaussian, formulas for approximately estimating the conditional means for z given that x is below or above the threshold (Eq. (2.7)). This was based on a formula for $E[z|x < thr]$ for the standard bivariate Gaussian by Mee and Owen (1983). The same authors also provided a formula to

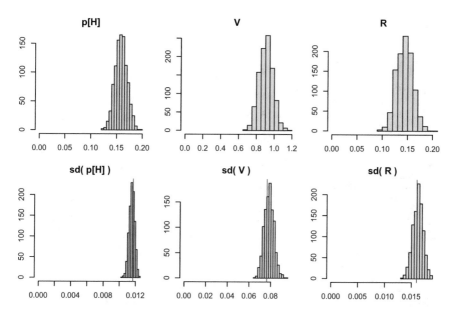

Fig. 4.5 PRAs on 1000 realisations from the same linear relationship between x and z. Top row: 1000 estimates for $p[H]$, V and R. Bottom row: 1000 uncertainty estimates. Vertical red lines indicate standard deviations of the top-row estimates

approximate the conditional variance for the same distribution: $Var[z|x < thr] = 1 + \rho\, thr\, E[z] - E[z]^2$. We can generalise their formula to all bivariate Gaussians and to $Var[z|x \geq thr]$ to derive approximate formulas for UQ in PRA:

APPRXOXIMATION FOR BIVARIATE GAUSSIAN p[x,z]:

$$Var[z|x < thr] \approx 1 + \rho\,(thr - E[x])\,(\mu_1 - E[z]) - (\mu_1 - E[z])^2, \qquad (4.5)$$

$$Var[z|x \geq thr] \approx 1 + \rho\,(thr - E[x])\,(\mu_2 - E[z]) - (\mu_2 - E[z])^2,$$

where $\mu_1 = E[z|x < thr]$ and $\mu_2 = E[z|x \geq thr]$ for which the approximations were given in Eq. (2.7). We encode the approximate PRA with UQ as follows:

```
PRA.UQAppr <- function( n=1e3, thr=0, mz.=mz, mx.=mx, Vz.=Vz, Vx.=Vx, r=rxz ) {

    Ez       <- mz.
    Ez_H     <- Ez_xbelowAppr(thr, mz., mx., Vz., Vx., r)
    Ez_notH  <- Ez_xaboveAppr(thr, mz., mx., Vz., Vx., r)
    pH       <- pnorm( thr, mx., sqrt(Vx.) ) ; nH <- n * pH
    V        <- Ez_notH - Ez_H
    R        <- Ez_notH - Ez
    # Or equivalently:
    # V       <- r * sqrt(Vx.*Vz.) * dnorm(thr, mx., sqrt(Vx.)) / (pH * (1-pH))
    # R       <- r * sqrt(Vx.*Vz.) * dnorm(thr, mx., sqrt(Vx.)) /       (1-pH)

    VarEz       <- Vz.                                             / n
    VarEz_H     <- Varz_xbelowAppr(thr, mz., mx., Vz., Vx., r) /  nH
    VarEz_notH  <- Varz_xaboveAppr(thr, mz., mx., Vz., Vx., r) / (n-nH)

     a  <- 1 + nH ; b <- 1 + n - nH
    s_pH <- sqrt( a*b/(a+b+1) ) / (a+b)
    s_V  <- sqrt( VarEz_notH + VarEz_H )
    s_R  <- sqrt( VarEz_notH + VarEz - 2 * VarEz_notH * (1-pH) )

    return( c(pH=pH,V=V,R=R,s_pH=s_pH,s_V=s_V,s_R=s_R) )
}
```

We now compare PRA with UQ for the bivariate normal using Monte Carlo sampling and PRA using the above approximate formulas (and Eqs. (2.7)–(2.8)). First the Monte Carlo result for a sample of $n = 10^6$ from our standard example of a bivariate Gaussian distribution:

```
>           pH              V              R         s_pH           s_V            s_R
> 0.1591340000 0.9053096781 0.1440655503 0.0003658011 0.0024676533 0.0005136846
```

And here is the PRA with UQ directly applied to the bivariate Gaussian using the approximation formulas:

```
>           pH              V              R         s_pH           s_V            s_R
> 0.1586552539 0.9063676236 0.1437999855 0.0003653544 0.0024737613 0.0005135115
```

We see that the results are similar.

Chapter 5
Density Estimation to Move from Sampling- to Distribution-Based PRA

Our approach to sampling-based single-threshold PRA with UQ in Chap. 4 was to take a collection of n data pairs (x, z), define a hazardous region H, and estimate $p[H]$, V and R as, respectively, n/n_H, $\overline{z_{\neg H}} - \overline{z_H}$ and $\overline{z_{\neg H}} - \overline{z}$. The approach was completed with UQ using Eqs. (4.1)–(4.4).

We now consider an alternative approach where we first fit a joint probability distribution $p[x, z]$ to the n data pairs (x, z). The idea is that $p[x, z]$ is expressed using known probability density functions (e.g. a Gaussian, a mixture of Gaussians, or any other known distribution), so that we can use Eqs. (2.2) or (2.3) to estimate the conditional expectations required for the PRA.

Let's begin with the example of the first 'linear' data set generated in Chap. 4 (top panel of Fig. 4.4). We fit a bivariate Gaussian distribution $N[m, V]$:

```
xz <- listxz[[1]] ; m <- colMeans(xz) ; V <- var(xz)
```

We now calculate the conditional expectations of Eq. (2.3) using the corresponding R-functions `Ez_xbelow` and `Ez_xabove` that we defined for bivariate Gaussian $p[x, z]$:

```
mx      <- m[1]    ; mz <- m[2]
Vx      <- V[1,1] ; Vz <- V[2,2] ; rxz <- V[1,2] / sqrt(Vx * Vz)
thr     <- -1
Ez      <- mz
Ez_xlo <- Ez_xbelow(thr=thr, mz.=mz, mx.=mx, Vz.=Vz, Vx.=Vx, r=rxz)
Ez_xhi <- Ez_xabove(thr=thr, mz.=mz, mx.=mx, Vz.=Vz, Vx.=Vx, r=rxz)
```

Supplementary Information The online version contains supplementary material available at https://doi.org/10.1007/978-3-031-16333-3_5

M. van Oijen, M. Brewer, *Probabilistic Risk Analysis and Bayesian Decision Theory*, SpringerBriefs in Statistics, https://doi.org/10.1007/978-3-031-16333-3_5

And that gives us the following 'distribution-from-sample'-based PRA:

```
V  <- Ez_xhi - Ez_xlo
R  <- Ez_xhi - Ez
pH <- R / V
```

The results are:

```
> PRA using density estimation and eqs for conditional expectations:
>   0.1543392 0.931134 0.1437105
```

UQ for this approach will have to include assessment of the reliability of the density estimation. This may require Bayesian density estimation (e.g. Shen et al. (2013)).

Note that even after the density estimation stage, the next steps are still not fully analytical because there are no closed-form solutions for conditional expectations when the condition is an inequality. Therefore our implementation of the equations in R-functions `Ez_xbelow` and `Ez_xabove` discretizes the domain of x.

The results that we just found differ slightly from what we found from inspecting the sample directly and using the observational means below and above the threshold (Eq. (3.1)):

```
>          pH          V          R       s_pH        s_V        s_R
> 0.15700000 1.00204916 0.15732172 0.01150752 0.07853827 0.01685975
```

Chapter 6
Copulas for Distribution-Based PRA

Our development of probabilistic risk analysis in this book centers on the joint probability distribution for an environmental variable x and a system variable z. This joint distribution, together with a decision on what values of x constitute hazardous conditions, is all the information we need to calculate risk and its decomposition into hazard probability and system vulnerability. The joint distribution is fully determined by its pdf $p[x, z]$, and equivalently by its joint cumulative distribution function F_{xz}. In the preceding chapters we showed how the PRA can be carried out on a sample from this joint distribution, either without or with a first step of density estimation (i.e. fitting a distribution). But there may be occasions where we have good information on the marginal distributions for x and z separately without having a good sample from the joint distribution. In such cases, we may want to use *copulas*, which are functions that map the marginal distributions F_x and F_z to F_{xz}. Sklar's Theorem (see e.g. Nelsen (2007)) guarantees that such a mapping is always possible: for every bivariate distribution we can write:

SKLAR's THEOREM:

$$F_{xz}(x, z) = C(F_x(x), F_z(z)),$$

(6.1)

where $C(., .)$ is a so-called copula function from the unit square $[0, 1]^2$ to the unit interval $[0, 1]$. [The theorem also holds for multivariate distributions of greater dimension than 2, but we shall not need that here.] If the marginal distribution functions are continuous, then only one unique copula maps a given pair of marginals to a given F_{xz}. Changing either the marginals or the copula leads to a different joint distribution.

Supplementary Information The online version contains supplementary material available at https://doi.org/10.1007/978-3-031-16333-3_6

M. van Oijen, M. Brewer, *Probabilistic Risk Analysis and Bayesian Decision Theory*, SpringerBriefs in Statistics, https://doi.org/10.1007/978-3-031-16333-3_6

In short, working with copulas allows us to decompose any joint distribution into its marginals on the one hand, and its correlation structure (embodied in the copula function C) on the other. Many types of copulas exist, each leading to a different pattern of correlation between the marginal variables.

6.1 Sampling from Copulas and Carrying out PRA

Let's study a copula in action. We assume $x \sim N[0, 1]$, $z \sim N[2, 1]$, and at first use a *Gaussian copula* which has only one parameter (a correlation coefficient) which we set as $\rho = 0.5$. For convenience, we use the R-package `copula` (Hofert et al., 2020) to implement this as follows:

```
cpN    <- normalCopula( param=0.5, dim=2 )
mvN.NN <- mvdc( cpN, margins = c("norm", "norm"),
                paramMargins = list( list( mean=0, sd=1 ),
                                     list( mean=2, sd=1 ) ) )
```

In the above code, we first chose a copula function, and then 'filled in the details' by choosing the marginals. This confirms that we can decide on the marginals independently from the correlation structure. So we could also sample from the copula before we choose our marginals. In the following code we do just that by first taking a sample from the copula and then taking a sample from the joint distribution determined by the combination of copula and marginals, and Fig. 6.1 shows the two samples plus two marginal histograms for x and z.

```
n                <- 1e3
sample.cpN    <- rCopula( n, cpN )
       Fx.N <- sample.cpN[,1]    ; Fz.N    <- sample.cpN[,2]
sample.mvN.NN <- rMvdc  ( n, mvN.NN )
       x.N.NN <- sample.mvN.NN[,1] ; z.N.NN <- sample.mvN.NN[,2]
```

With these choices of Gaussian copula and Gaussian marginals, the joint distribution is simply a bivariate Gaussian, and we could have studied that without the copula-apparatus. But the copula allows us to change the marginals to define new joint distributions.

To show this, we repeat the sampling from the same copula but change one of the marginal distributions: we replace the Gaussian for z with a Gamma-distribution $z \sim \Gamma[4, 2]$. This distribution has a mean equal to 2 and a variance equal to 1, which are the same values as the Gaussian that we had before. The results when

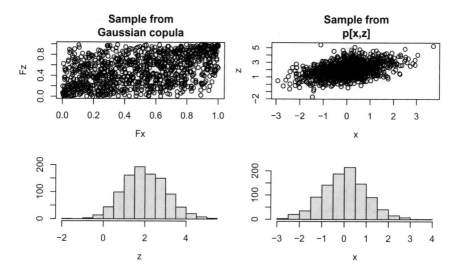

Fig. 6.1 Top left: sample from a Gaussian copula with correlation parameter $\rho = 0.5$. Top right: sample from the joint distribution determined by this copula when the marginals for x and z are N[0,1] and N[2,1]. Bottom row: marginal samples

using this new marginal are shown in Fig. 6.2, where we see that quite different joint distributions are produced from the same copula.

```
mvN.NG         <- mvdc( cpN, margins = c("norm", "gamma"),
                        paramMargins = list( list( mean =0, sd   =1 ),
                                             list( shape=4, scale=2 ) ) )
sample.mvN.NG <- rMvdc( n, mvN.NG )
        x.N.NG <- sample.mvN.NG[,1] ; z.N.NG <- sample.mvN.NG[,2]
```

Let's now carry out a PRA on both samples. Here are the results from PRA on the first sample, from the copula with both marginals being Gaussian:

```
>    pH    V    R  s_pH   s_V   s_R
> 0.150 0.820 0.120 0.011 0.084 0.016
```

And here are the results for the second sample, where the marginal for z was replaced by a Gamma distribution:

```
>    pH    V    R  s_pH   s_V   s_R
> 0.160 3.500 0.580 0.012 0.240 0.057
```

We see that hazard probabilities are about the same for both samples, as they should be because we did not change $p[x]$. But with the right-skewed Gamma for $p[z]$ we find much higher values of system vulnerability and thus risk.

Let's now keep the same pair of Gaussian and Gamma marginals for x and z but combine them with a different copula. This time we choose a *t-copula*, with

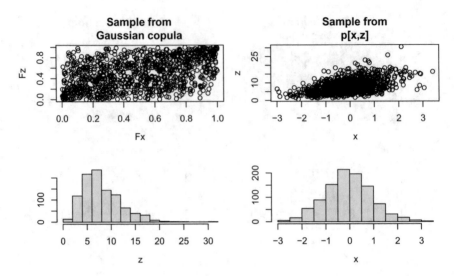

Fig. 6.2 Sampling from a Gaussian copula with correlation parameter $\rho = 0.5$ combined with N[0,1] and Gamma[4,2] marginals for x and z

as parameters $\rho = 0.5$ and one degree of freedom df $= 1$. With this low value for df the t-distribution has much heavier tails than the Gaussian. We carry out the sampling and the PRA as above for this combination of copula and marginals. The samples are shown in Fig. 6.3, and the PRA results are as follows:

```
cpt <- tCopula( param=0.5, df=1 )


>     pH      V      R   s_pH    s_V    s_R
> 0.150  1.600  0.240  0.011  0.430  0.067
```

We see that the PRA-results are again different from what we found before, there is some reduction in vulnerability and risk. However, in this case the choice of copula had slightly less impact than the choice of marginals. This is not a general rule, so we always need to select our copula carefully, which we discuss next.

6.2 Copula Selection

When we have a sample of data $\{(x_i, z_i)\}$, we can use a semi-Bayesian approach to copula-selection which is built into the R-package VineCopula and which uses information criteria (AIC or BIC can be chosen) to select the best copula and

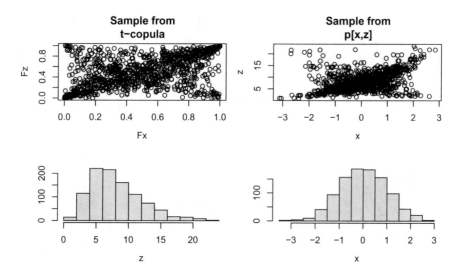

Fig. 6.3 Sampling from a t-copula with correlation parameter $\rho = 0.5$ and $df = 1$ combined with N[0,1] and Gamma[4,2] marginals for x and z

parameterise it. Here is the code and the results for all three combinations of copula + marginals that we studied above:

```
fitC <- function(x,z){ BiCopSelect( ecdf(x)(x)*n/(n+1), ecdf(z)(z)*n/(n+1),
                          sel="BIC" ) }
fitC( x.N.NN, z.N.NN )
> Bivariate copula: Gaussian (par = 0.44, tau = 0.29)
fitC( x.N.NG, z.N.NG )
> Bivariate copula: Gaussian (par = 0.52, tau = 0.34)
fitC( x.t.NG, z.t.NG )
> Bivariate copula: t (par = 0.54, par2 = 2, tau = 0.36)
```

We see that in each of the three examples, the correct copula family was selected (i.e. the one that was used to generate the samples in the first place) with a correlation parameter close to 0.5. Also, for the t-copula a small value of $df = 2$ was estimated, close to the value equal to 1 that was used to generate the sample.

We conclude this chapter by plotting samples from a number of different copulas and parameter settings to show that they allow for a wide range of different correlation structures (Fig. 6.4). Note that the choice of copula determines whether correlations between x and z are strongest in the lower or upper tail.

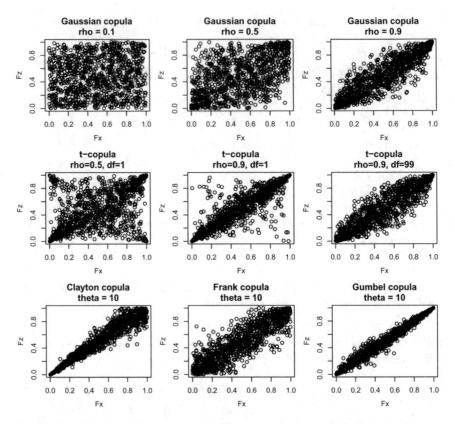

Fig. 6.4 Sampling from different copula families and parameter settings. Top row: Gaussian copulas. Middle row: t-copulas. Bottom row: Clayton, Frank and Gumbel copulas

6.3 Using Copulas in PRA

Copulas are commonly used in financial risk analysis (e.g. Embrechts et al. (2003) and Nguyen-Huy et al. (2018)), but they are increasingly used in other areas too, such as environmental risk management (e.g. Li et al. (2020), Schölzel and Friederichs (2008), Laux et al. (2011), Jane et al. (2018), and Salvadori et al. (2018)). Genest and Favre (2007) provide a simple introduction to copulas and discuss choosing between 20 copula-families for modelling correlations between annual peak and volume of river flow.

In this chapter, we focused on bivariate copulas for F_{xz}. However, a natural extension would be to increase the dimension of the environmental variable, e.g. by having x_1 be precipitation and x_2 temperature. That would lead to trivariate copulas which does not pose any problems.

Bayesian selection of copulas is still in its infancy (Huard et al., 2006; Rosen & Thompson, 2015) so full uncertainty quantification is not yet straightforward. The PRA-uncertainties for $p[H]$, V and R that we reported in this chapter therefore do not account for uncertainty in copula selection or parameter estimation. Steps toward more comprehensive Bayesian UQ are provided in the following chapter.

Chapter 7
Bayesian Model-Based PRA

In practice, given a particular data set we will want to model the relationship between outcome/response variables and associated explanatory variables. We can then use this model to conduct our PRA. We will illustrate this using the existing linear (bivariate Gaussian) and nonlinear examples.

We take a fully Bayesian approach. That means that (1) we find a suitable model for the given data, (2) assign prior probability distributions to the model's parameters and (3) use Bayes' Theorem to obtain an estimate of the joint posterior distribution for the parameters (Bayes, 1763; Van Oijen, 2020). We can then apply a PRA to the model variables, and obtain estimates of the full posterior distributions of quantities like V and R too. We take a sampling approach, using MCMC where necessary, or plain Monte Carlo sampling where not.

We will use the R package Nimble for our MCMC, as this allows computation to be performed within R (not requiring us to call external software such as WinBUGS or JAGS) for simplicity and robustness.

7.1 Linear Example: Full Bayesian PRA with Uncertainty

For the linear bivariate Gaussian example, we generate x and z as before. A suitable model for these data would be a straight-line linear regression:

$$z_i = \alpha + \beta x_i + \epsilon_i \quad \forall i = 1, 2, \ldots, n \tag{7.1}$$

and where $\epsilon_i \sim N(0, \sigma^2)$. We fit this model in Nimble using the following code.

Supplementary Information The online version contains supplementary material available at https://doi.org/10.1007/978-3-031-16333-3_7

```
Model1.Code <- nimbleCode({
  lm.alpha.centred   ~ dnorm ( 0, sd=100 )
  lm.alpha          <- lm.alpha.centred - lm.beta*xmean
  lm.beta            ~ dnorm ( 0, sd=100 )
  lm.tau             ~ dgamma( 0.01, 0.01 )
  lm.sigma          <- 1 / sqrt(lm.tau)
  xmean             <- mean( x[1:ndata] )
  for(i in 1:ndata){
    lm.mu[i] <- lm.alpha.centred + lm.beta*(x[i]-xmean)
    z[i]       ~ dnorm( lm.mu[i], sd=lm.sigma )
  }
} )
Model1.Constants <- list( ndata=length(x), x=x )
Model1.Data        <- list( z=z )
Model1.Nimble     <- nimbleModel ( Model1.Code, constants=Model1.Constants,
                                                  data=Model1.Data )
Model1.Comp       <- compileNimble( Model1.Nimble )
Model1.Conf       <- configureMCMC( Model1.Nimble, print=F )
Model1.Conf$addMonitors( c("lm.alpha", "lm.sigma"), print=F )
Model1.MCMC       <- buildMCMC    ( Model1.Conf )
Model1.MCMC.Comp <- compileNimble( Model1.MCMC )
```

7.1.1 Checking the MCMC

We can plot traces for checking convergence of the MCMC sampling (Fig. 7.1), and
do a sense check on the results from the MCMC from a direct linear regression in R
using the `lm()` function.

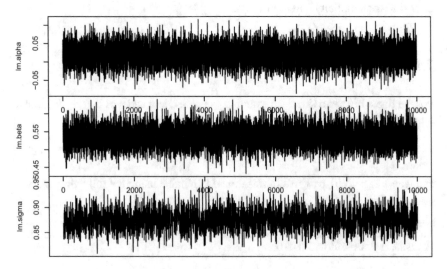

Fig. 7.1 Parameter trace plots generated by Nimble for the linear example

```
>       Min.   1st Qu.    Median     Mean   3rd Qu.       Max.
> -0.085815  0.001992  0.021063  0.020649  0.039349  0.115977
>     Min. 1st Qu.  Median    Mean 3rd Qu.     Max.
>   0.4333  0.5171  0.5359  0.5361  0.5548  0.6405
>     Min. 1st Qu.  Median    Mean 3rd Qu.     Max.
>   0.8085  0.8621  0.8754  0.8757  0.8895  0.9559
>
> Call:
> lm(formula = z ~ x)
>
> Residuals:
>      Min       1Q   Median       3Q      Max
> -3.01340 -0.58434 -0.01747  0.59079  2.78595
>
> Coefficients:
>              Estimate Std. Error t value Pr(>|t|)
> (Intercept)  0.02052    0.02766   0.742    0.458
> x            0.53578    0.02808  19.080   <2e-16 ***
> ---
> Signif. codes:  0 '***' 0.001 '**' 0.01 '*' 0.05 '.' 0.1 ' ' 1
>
> Residual standard error: 0.8746 on 998 degrees of freedom
> Multiple R-squared:  0.2673,  Adjusted R-squared:  0.2665
> F-statistic:   364 on 1 and 998 DF,  p-value: < 2.2e-16
```

7.1.2 PRA

It is possible to run the linear regression model analysis generating samples from the joint posterior distributions of all model parameters *at the same time as* the PRA assessment; here for illustration we simply obtain samples from the resulting full posterior distributions for V and R; these quantities are calculated directly on samples from the fitted model, so can be calculated to arbitrary accuracy. Note that the samples obtained from the posteriors for V and R can be used directly to provide (credible) interval estimates (and standard errors).

We have the choice of using either the samples from the full posterior distribution for the linear regression model parameters (that is, α, β and σ) or the estimates (posterior samples means) when generating samples from the fitted model; the former allows for the uncertainty in estimating the regression model, should that be desired.

As before, we investigate the values of V and R with respect to the threshold values, with associated uncertainty: see Fig. 7.2. Compare this with our earlier study of this linear example where we carried out distribution-based PRA for this linear example but without UQ (Fig. 2.3).

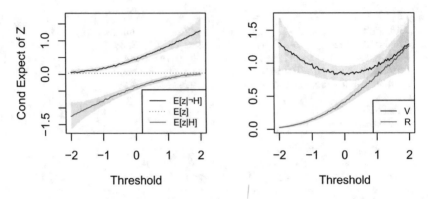

Fig. 7.2 PRA on linearly related x and z, with UQ following Bayesian modelling with Nimble

7.2 Nonlinear Example: Full Bayesian PRA with Uncertainty

We repeat the above analysis for the nonlinear example. Here we will need a slightly more complex regression model; for illustration we use the model used to generate the data, although in reality this will not exist—so model choice is a further source of uncertainty.

```
n <- 1e3 ; sz <- 0.1
x <- runif( n, 0, 3 ) ; ez <- rnorm( n, 0, sz) ; z <- 1-exp(-x) + ez
Model1.Code <- nimbleCode({
  lm.alpha  ~ dnorm( 0, sd=100 )
  lm.beta   ~ dnorm( 0, sd=100 )
  lm.tau    ~ dgamma( 0.01, 0.01 )
  lm.sigma <- 1 / sqrt(lm.tau)
  for(i in 1:ndata){
    lm.mu[i] <- lm.alpha + lm.beta*exp(-x[i])
    z[i]      ~ dnorm( lm.mu[i], sd=lm.sigma )
  }
} )
```

We now run the MCMC as we did in the previous example for the linear model, not showing code and results for checking convergence. We then carry out PRA with UQ as before and show the results in Fig. 7.3. Note the similarity with the results that we found before using sampling without Bayesian modelling of the relationship between x and z (see the rightmost panels in Fig. 4.1).

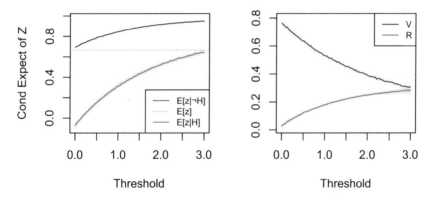

Fig. 7.3 PRA on nonlinearly related x and z, with UQ following Bayesian modelling with Nimble

7.3   Advantages of the Bayesian Modelling Approach

Whenever we use the approach taken in this chapter, we always begin by fitting a model $z = f(x; \theta) + \epsilon$, with uncertain parameters θ and uncertain model error ϵ. We then calibrate the model in a Bayesian way which allows quantification of prior uncertainties and the derivation of posterior uncertainties that drive the PRA. So this approach allows us to build in uncertainty in a formal, modelled way, of any quantity we wish to study, including V and R. We can therefore cope with situations of missing data, or where expert opinion is all we have. Non-parametric densities can be used, which Nimble can handle.

Note that if we do not provide a model for the data, as in the previous chapters, the implicit assumption is that the data set *is* the model, which is effectively what non-parametric bootstrapping is doing, for example.

Chapter 8
Sampling-Based Multi-Threshold PRA: Gaussian Linear Example

In this section, we carry out multi-threshold PRA which distinguishes multiple levels of hazard, such that H is the union of $H_1, .. H_n$. The relevant Eqs. (1.4) and (1.5) were already shown in Chap. 1. We begin by defining a new R-function for PRA that takes (besides a sample of x and z values) a vector of threshold-values:

```
PRAn <- function( x, z, thr=-1:1 ) {
  n   <- length(z) ; nthr <- length(thr)
  H   <- vector("list",nthr)
  nH <- Ez_H <- pH <- V <- R <- rep(NA,nthr)

  H[[1]] <- which( x < thr[1] ) ; nH[1] <- length(H[[1]])
  for(i in 2:nthr) {
    H[[i]] <- which( thr[i-1] <= x & x < thr[i]) ; nH[i] <- length(H[[i]]) }

  H.all   <- NULL ; for(i in 1:nthr) { H.all <- c( H.all, H[[i]] ) }
  Ez_notH <- mean( z[-H.all] )

  for(i in 1:nthr) {
    Ez_H[i] <- mean( z[ H[[i]] ] )
    pH[i]   <- nH[i] / n
    V[i]    <- Ez_notH - Ez_H[i]
    R[i]    <- pH[i] * V[i] }

  R.sum  <- sum(R)
  pH.sum <- sum(pH)
  V.wsum <- R.sum / pH.sum
  return( list( pH.sum=pH.sum, V.wsum=V.wsum, R.sum=R.sum,
                pH   =pH    , V   =V  , R    =R    ) ) }
```

Supplementary Information The online version contains supplementary material available at https://doi.org/10.1007/978-3-031-16333-3_8

M. van Oijen, M. Brewer, *Probabilistic Risk Analysis and Bayesian Decision Theory*, SpringerBriefs in Statistics, https://doi.org/10.1007/978-3-031-16333-3_8

This function implements Eqs. (1.4) as well as (1.5). So it not only returns the PRA-terms for each of the n different hazard levels but also the overall terms.

We continue with the linear data (bivariate Gaussian) example. Here is our multi-threshold PRA function in action on these data with a threshold-vector that has only 2 entries. That represents a PRA which distinguishes the two categories of 'severe' and 'moderate' hazardous conditions.

```
thr <- -1:-0 ; pran <- PRAn(x, z, thr)
```

```
> Overall values: pH.sum = 0.502 ; V.wsum = 0.8482974 ; R.sum = 0.4258453
> Vector values pH: 0.17 0.332
> Vector values V : 1.257536 0.6387476
> Vector values R : 0.2137811 0.2120642
```

Note that the overall values are simply the sums of the vector values (weighted by relative hazard probabilities in the case of V), as we showed in Eq. (1.5).

Now we test our function for the case of four different threshold-levels.

```
thr  <- -3:0 ; pran <- PRAn(x, z, thr)
```

```
> Overall values: pH.sum = 0.502 ; V.wsum = 0.8482974 ; R.sum = 0.4258453
> Vector values pH: 0.003 0.023 0.144 0.332
> Vector values V : 3.094876 1.686693 1.150712 0.6387476
> Vector values R : 0.009284628 0.03879395 0.1657025 0.2120642
```

Finally, we use a very long threshold-vector, of 31 equidistant values in the interval $[-2, 1]$. We take a large sample from (x, z) so that there will be enough observations in every interval to produce smooth plots.

```
n    <- 1e5 ; xz <- rmvnorm( n, mxz, Sxz ) ; x <- xz[,1] ; z <- xz[,2]
thr <- seq(-2,1,0.1) ; pran <- PRAn (x, z, thr)
```

Because of the large number of hazard-levels, this time we do not give tables of results but barplots (Fig. 8.1):

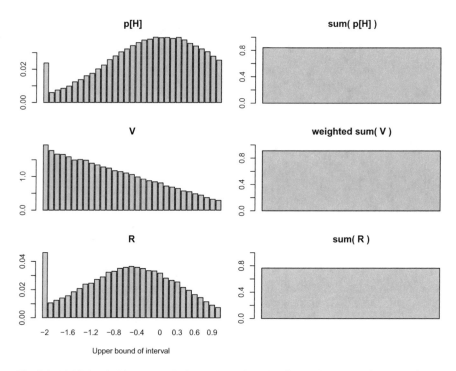

Fig. 8.1 Multi-threshold PRA applied to a large Gaussian linear data set. Left: results for 31 hazard-levels. Right: overall (summed) values for all hazard levels combined

Chapter 9
Distribution-Based Continuous PRA: Gaussian Linear Example

We now turn to continuous PRA, which can be viewed as the limit of multi-threshold PRA when the number of thresholds goes to infinity. We already showed the equations for continuous PRA above (Eqs. (1.6) and (1.7)), and implement this form of PRA now for the same bivariate Gaussian that we studied in previous sections. We accept the Gaussian distribution as given, so we can apply distribution-based PRA:

```
p <- px # Gaussian density function as defined above
  mx   <- mz <- 0 ; rxz <- 0.5
  Ez_x <- function(x){ mz + (x-mx)*rxz }
v <- function(x,thr=0) { Ez_xabove(thr) - Ez_x(x) }
r <- function(x,thr=0) { p(x) * v(x,thr) }

thr   <- 1
p.seq <- p(x.seq) ; v.seq <- v(x.seq,thr) ; r.seq <- r(x.seq,thr)
```

The results are shown in Fig. 9.1. As expected, the continuous curves for $p[x]$, $v(x)$ and $r(x)$ of the continuous PRA closely resemble the barplots for multi-threshold PRA of Fig. 8.1 because of the high number of hazard-levels that we used there [Note that the vertical scales for $p[H]$ and R in our multi-threshold PRA are ten times shorter than those for $p[x]$ and $r(x)$ in our continuous PRA because the former are integrals over hazard-classes that were chosen to be 0.1 unit wide.].

Supplementary Information The online version contains supplementary material available at https://doi.org/10.1007/978-3-031-16333-3_9

M. van Oijen, M. Brewer, *Probabilistic Risk Analysis and Bayesian Decision Theory*, SpringerBriefs in Statistics, https://doi.org/10.1007/978-3-031-16333-3_9

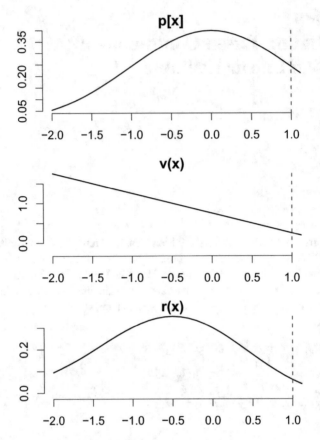

Fig. 9.1 Continuous PRA applied to a bivariate Gaussian dsistribution

Chapter 10
Categorical PRA with Other Splits than for Threshold-Levels: Spatio-Temporal Example

In multi-threshold PRA, we split up the hazardous region H (defined by some highest threshold-value) into a range of intervals for the environmental variable x. But other ways of splitting up H can be envisaged too. We may for example think of how lag-effects and cumulative effects of hazards affect the impact of drought.

The importance of such legacy effects of forest drought in later years has been reported by various authors (Borghetti et al., 2020; Brodribb et al., 2020; Brun et al., 2020; Gessler et al., 2020; Guérin et al., 2020; Kannenberg et al., 2020; Khoury & Coomes, 2020; Schuldt et al., 2020; Szejner et al., 2020). For example, Pappas et al. (2020) carried out an analysis of 'statistical memory' (in this case decay of disturbance-induced variability) and found that growth remained perturbed longer than water use, and more so in Norway spruce than in European larch. A relevant distinction could be whether a drought in 1 year is followed by another drought, or alternatively by a non-hazardous year in which the vegetation can recover. That would mean distinguishing two categories of drought, and we implement that example in this chapter.

Other possibilities for *categorical PRA* are distinguishing different types of hazard (e.g. drought, flooding, infestation, etc.) whose union would be the overall hazardous region and where we can quantify the contribution of the different hazard types to overall risk.

We introduce another novelty in this chapter: spatially distributed risk analysis in which we carry out a PRA for different locations within a larger area. We investigate how the prevalence and impact of the two categories of drought (stand-alone droughts vs. droughts that follow an earlier one) vary in this area. We begin by generating a (virtual) spatio-temporal data set $\{x(s, t), z(s, t)\}$. We shall then

Supplementary Information The online version contains supplementary material available at https://doi.org/10.1007/978-3-031-16333-3_10

M. van Oijen, M. Brewer, *Probabilistic Risk Analysis and Bayesian Decision Theory*, SpringerBriefs in Statistics, https://doi.org/10.1007/978-3-031-16333-3_10

first analyse that data set as before, distinguishing just a single category of drought, before finally showing the two-category approach.

10.1 Spatio-Temporal Environmental Data: $x(s, t)$

We assume a zero mean for x and define a simple function for 'predicting' x-values at new locations conditional on the x-values that we already have at other locations or earlier. Our implementation is a stochastic process $x(s, t)$ which combines a Gaussian Process (GP) in space and an autoregressive process (AR(1)) in time.

```
GP.AR <- function( s0, s, x, Vx.s, phi, x0past=0, Vx.t=0, alpha=0 ) {
  ds  <- as.matrix( dist(s) )
  rx  <- exp( -ds/phi )
  ds0 <- sapply(1:length(x),function(i){dist(rbind(s0,s[i,]))})
  r0  <- exp( -ds0/phi )
  m0  <- t(r0) %*% solve(rx) %*% x + alpha * x0past
  V0  <- Vx.s * (1 - t(r0) %*% solve(rx) %*% r0 ) + Vx.t
  return( c( m0=m0, V0=V0 ) ) }
```

We want to build up one realisation of our spatio-temporal model for a rectangular area of $ns = ns1 \times ns2$ cells and for nt time steps. We begin by defining dimensions, variances and correlation lengths:

```
ns1 <- 8 ; ns2 <- 8 ; nt <- 9
xst <- array( NA, dim=c(ns1,ns2,nt) )

Vx.s <- 0.5 ; phi   <- 1
Vx.t <- 0.5 ; alpha <- 0.5
```

We generate one realisation of our spatiotemporal model for our environmental variable $x(s, t)$ using an iterative algorithm that starts at cell (1,1) at t=1 and then fills the other cells row by row and time step by time step. We normalise the generated data to the interval [0,1]. The resulting maps of $x(s, t)$ are shown in Fig. 10.1.

At each time step we calculate a variogram to show spatial correlations in our data, as shown in Fig. 10.2. Clearly, the Gaussian Process has provided significant correlation up to a distance of about six cells away.

Temporal correlation is shown in Fig. 10.3. We see that the AR(1) process has ensured that the values of $x(s, t)$ in each cell are strongly correlated with the values the time step before, i.e. $x(s, t - 1)$.

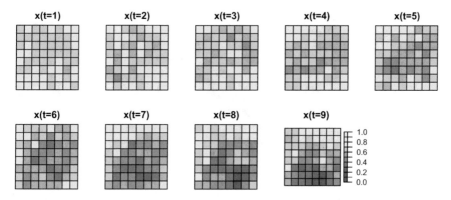

Fig. 10.1 Evolution of the environmental variable $x(s, t)$ over time

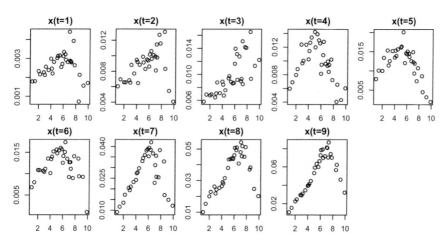

Fig. 10.2 Spatial variograms for $x(z, t)$

10.2 Spatio-Temporal System Data: $z(s, t)$

We assume a deterministic nonlinear system response where the response variable $z(t)$ is a logistic function of a weighted sum of $x(t)$ and $x(t - 1)$:

```
fz  <- function( x, xpast=1, k=10 ) {
  1 / (1 + exp( -k * (x + xpast/2 - 0.5 ) ) ) }
```

We normalise $z(s, t)$ to the interval $[0, 1]$ and plot its evolution over time in Fig. 10.4.

Figure 10.5 summarizes how our response function works out for the whole data set, i.e. it shows in one scatterplot the data points $(x(s, t), z(s, t))$ that we generated for all locations and all times. The figure shows that there is conditional

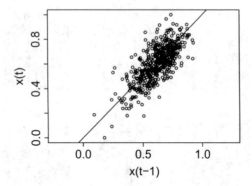

Fig. 10.3 Temporal correlation of the environmental variable

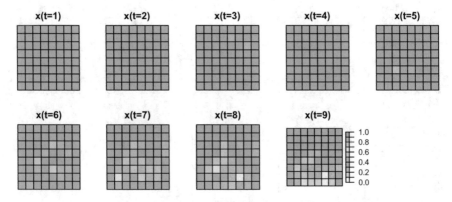

Fig. 10.4 Evolution of the response variable $z(s, t)$ over time

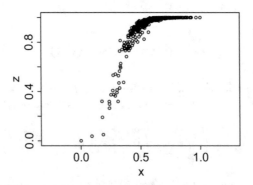

Fig. 10.5 Responses of z to x for all locations and times

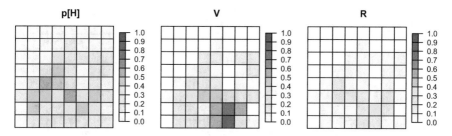

Fig. 10.6 PRAs for all cells in a square region. Each of the 64 PRAs was based on a single cell's time series of (x, z)

variation in the vertical direction (positive $Var[z(t)|x(t)]$) which is not because of a stochastic response function (as our model has a deterministic response) but because of variation in $x(t-1)$. Our response function produces lower values for z when there was a drought also in the preceding year.

10.3   Single-Category Single-Threshold PRA for the Spatio-Temporal Data

We define the hazardous region as the environmental variable x being less than its 0.1587 quantile (which for a Gaussian distribution would be one standard deviation below the mean).

```
thr.xst <- quantile( xst, pnorm(-1) )
```

We then carry out a separate PRA for each cell, using its time series of x and z, and show the results in Fig. 10.6. This first spatially distributed single-threshold PRA does not yet distinguish different categories of drought. The next section will finally introduce the two drought categories that we mentioned at the beginning of this chapter.

10.4   Two-Category Single-Threshold PRA for Spatio-Temporal Data

We now modify the PRA-calculation to distinguish two categories of drought: drought preceded or not preceded by drought in the time step before.

The results of the 2-category PRAs for all grid cells are shown in Fig. 10.7. We see that for our virtual data set the first category of droughts (those preceded by a drought in the time step before) are more frequent and the system is more vulnerable

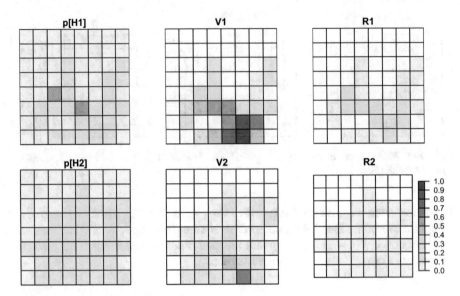

Fig. 10.7 Two-category PRAs for all cells in a square region. Top row: category 1 droughts (preceded by drought in the time step before). Bottom row: category 2 droughts (not preceded by drought)

to them, so the risks associated with such 'second droughts' are much larger than those associated with 'first droughts.'

Chapter 11
Three-Component PRA

So far we have discussed theory for two-component PRA, where $R = p[H] \times V$. In such PRA, risk R and vulnerability V must be expressed in the same units because $p[H]$ is a dimensionless probability. For example, in forestry both R and V would typically be quantified in units of productivity such as $m^3 m^{-2} y^{-1}$. These units imply that R and V are *intensive* properties of the system, as they do not account for the size of the forest that is at risk.

We now consider extending the risk decomposition to three components by the addition of a term for *exposure*, so that $R = p[H] \times Q \times V$, where we denote exposure as Q (rather than E) to avoid confusion with the symbol for mathematical expectation.

Three-component PRA is useful when we want to include the size of the system at risk in the analysis. Q could for example be defined as the area of forest or the number of trees exposed to a hazard. If we choose the former by expressing Q in units of m^2 and we keep the original intensive definition of V, then R becomes an *extensive* property: the expected total of the loss for the whole forest area in $m^3 y^{-1}$.

To introduce three-component PRA, we shall be using the same virtual spatio-temporal data set as in the preceding chapter.

11.1   Three-Component PRA for Spatio-Temporal Data

We define exposure as the number of cells in the region covered by our data set (8×8 cells) that experience drought at least once during their whole time series. So Q would be equal to all cells in the region if drought occurs everywhere occasionally,

Supplementary Information The online version contains supplementary material available at https://doi.org/10.1007/978-3-031-16333-3_11

but it can also be a smaller number. In our example of a region with 64 cells, $Q \in$ {0, 1, .., 64}.

Three-component PRA is not applied to individual cells in a region, but to the region as a whole. So whereas before we carried out 64 two-component PRAs, we now carry out just one three-component PRA. This is done in three steps:

1. Identify and count the 'exposed' cells in the region, giving us Q,
2. Carry out 2-component PRA on the exposed subregion, giving us $p[H]$ and $R_{intensive}$,
3. Calculate expected loss for the whole region as $R_{extensive} = Q \times R_{intensive}$.

Let's apply this algorithm to our spatio-temporal example.

STEP 1.   Keeping the same x-threshold as before (i.e. the 0.1587 quantile of x) and the same virtual data set, we find that in 37 of the 64 cells there is at least one time step with drought, so $Q = 37$.

STEP 2.   Ignoring the non-exposed cells where drought never happened, and lumping all the data from the 37 exposed cells together, we carry out one two-component PRA.

STEP 3.   Combining the results from the first two steps, we calculate $R_{extensive}$:

```
> Three-component PRA:
>     Q = 37 ; pH = 0.2762763 ; V = 0.2604741
>     Rintensive = 0.07196282 ; Rextensive = 2.662624
```

That completes our example of three-component PRA.

11.2   Country-Wide Application of Three-Component PRA

When applying this method to a large area such as Scotland or the UK, we can imagine subdividing the country in cells of $1 \times 1\,km^2$ which are then grouped in blocks of 8×8 cells. The three-component PRA could then be applied to each block, thereby generating a low-resolution map of how Q, $p[H]$, and V vary across the country. Because not all blocks will have the same number of cells (e.g. coastal blocks) we may then want to express exposure Q as the fraction (rather than the number) of cells that experience drought at least once.

• We show an example of such country-wide 3-component PRA in Chap. 18.

11.3   UQ for Three-Component PRA

Uncertainty quantification for three-component PRA is more complicated than for two-component PRA. It may be approached in two steps: (1) quantify the uncertainty of $R_{intensive} = p[H] \times V$ as before, (2) quantify the uncertainty of

$R_{extensive} = R_{intensive} \times Q$ using the standard equation for (the square root of) the variance of a product of independent random variables:

$$\sigma_{R_e R_i} = \sqrt{\sigma_{R_e}^2 \sigma_{R_i}^2 + \sigma_{R_e}^2 E[R_i]^2 + \sigma_{R_i}^2 E[R_e]^2}. \tag{11.1}$$

Chapter 12
Introduction to Bayesian Decision Theory (BDT)

This chapter provides a simple introduction to Bayesian decision theory (BDT) and its core idea: *maximising the expectation for utility*. We keep the mathematics to a minimum and develop the ideas using a general graphical model for decision-making, referring to the literature for details.

BDT is a theory for optimal decision-making under conditions of uncertainty (Berger, 1985; Lindley, 2000, 1991; Mazumder, 2003; Parmigiani & Inoue, 2009; Williams & Hooten, 2016). The theory has been recommended for many applications, e.g. model comparison (Vehtari & Ojanen, 2012), plant breeding (Villar-Hernández et al., 2018), the design of adaptive monitoring programmes (Williams & Hooten, 2016) and natural resource management (Dorazio & Johnson, 2003). Strong arguments for the use of BDT have been given, but the approach has not found much application in the environmental sciences or landscape management. Two reasons for this are the perceived complexity of the approach (Bordley & Pollock, 2009) and its computational demand. We show here that the method is actually straightforward, and we show how Markov Chain Monte Carlo sampling (MCMC) can be used in the computations. We begin with a graphical introduction to the theory.

The *graphical model* (GM) of Fig. 12.1 depicts the general joint probability distribution for decision-making under uncertainty.

A graphical model, also called a *probabilistic network*, is a representation of a joint probability distribution (Van Oijen, 2020, Chap. 15). A GM has two parts: (1) a graph with nodes connected by edges, (2) information about the nodes. The graph is just the visible part of the model. GMs do not represent a special kind of statistical model, they are just helpful tools for analysing joint probability distributions. Every joint distribution, continuous or discrete, can be represented by a GM.

Supplementary Information The online version contains supplementary material available at https://doi.org/10.1007/978-3-031-16333-3_12

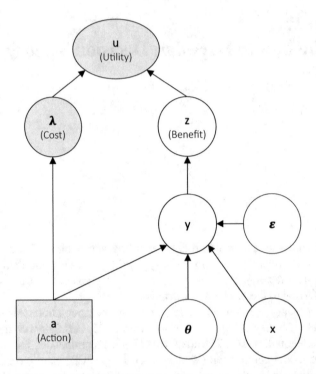

Fig. 12.1 A graphical model for Bayesian decision theory. See text for explanation of symbols

The GM of Fig. 12.1 aims to clarify how we quantify the *utility* $u(a, x)$. Neither the decision maker's *actions a* nor the *environmental conditions x* directly affect u. Instead, the utility is the difference between the *benefits z* from our system's *performance y* and the *costs* λ of the actions. For example, in forestry the performance could be wood production leading to benefits in the form of money received and the action could be irrigation at a certain cost.

The system performance y depends on the actions a, which are to be decided, and the environmental conditions x, which are not under human control. Our conditional probability distribution for y will depend on *model prediction* $f(x, a, \theta)$ which accounts for uncertainty about parameter values (θ) and may be biased because of *model structural error* ϵ.

Uncertainty about parameter values may be reduced by *Bayesian calibration*. In terms of our graphical model, as applied to forestry, that would mean that we require observations on forest growth y under known conditions x and actions a. Bayes' Theorem (Bayes, 1763) then tells us how these data change the joint probability distribution for the parameters.

12.1 Example of BDT in Action

The graphical model of Fig. 12.1 represents our joint distribution by showing the uncertain variables and parameters and their relationships, but it does not specify the exact nature of the dependencies. So we now give an example where we make the dependencies explicit. Note that this will be a toy example with less complexity than practical decision problems but with the same key elements. We make the following simplifying assumptions:

- All variables and parameters take values on a continuous scale.
- Only the error ϵ can be negative.
- Costs are proportional to the action: $\lambda = k_a\, a$, where k_a is the price paid for one unit of a.
- Benefits are proportional to the production y: $z = k_y\, y$, where k_y is the benefit received for one unit of y.
- y is a deterministic function of actions, environmental conditions and parameters, plus an uncertain error: $y = f(a, x, \theta) + \epsilon$.
- f can be nonlinear.
- Past observations on production under different conditions may provide information about the parameters of f by means of Bayes' Theorem: $p[\theta | x_{past}, y_{past}] \propto p[\theta]\, p[y_{past} | x_{past}, \theta]$.

Using these assumptions, we now write an R-function that calculates the utility u as a function of the values of the various variables and parameters:

```
u <- function( a, x, f, t, e, ka, ky ) {
    y        <- f(a,x,t) + e
    cost     <- ka * a
    benefit  <- ky * y
    return( benefit - cost ) }
```

Let's take the example of a negative exponential performance function: $f(a, x, \theta) = \theta(1 - e^{-a-x})$ and choose some default values for the function arguments. Utility is then a concave function of action a, as shown in Fig. 12.2.

```
fy <- function(a,x,t) { t * (1-exp(-a-x)) }
fu <- function( a, x=1, t=1, e=0, ka=0.2, ky=1 ) {
           u( a, x, f=fy, t, e, ka, ky) }
```

If we were certain that our default settings of all variables and parameters were correct, then the decision problem would be a simple matter of identifying the value of action a that maximises the utility in Fig. 12.2. But we do have uncertainties, so the Bayesian decision problem is to find the value of a that maximises the *conditional expectation for utility* $E[u|a]$ that we calculate by integrating out the uncertainties. (Henceforth we take the conditioning on a as understood and

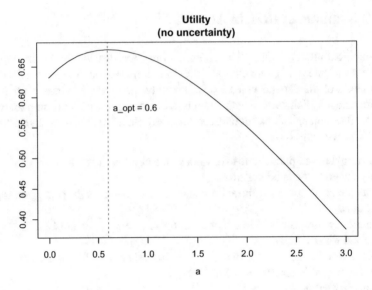

Fig. 12.2 Utility as a function of action a for a negative exponential performance function and linear cost and benefit functions

write $E[u]$.) Let's show that for an example. We assign the following probability distributions:

$$
\begin{aligned}
x &\sim N[1, 1], \\
t &\sim N[1, 0.5], \\
e &\sim N[0, 1], \\
ka &\sim U[0.1, 0.3], \\
ky &\sim U[0.5, 1.5].
\end{aligned}
\tag{12.1}
$$

The analysis of this decision problem with uncertainty is shown in the middle panel of Fig. 12.3. We see that the optimum action is now 1.1, which is larger than it was without uncertainty. And if we increase the uncertainty by a factor 1.5, then the optimum action increases even further (right panel of Fig. 12.3). Reducing the uncertainty by the same factor reduces the optimum to 0.8 as shown in the left panel.

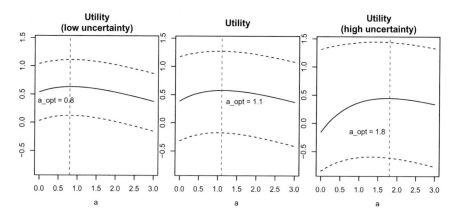

Fig. 12.3 Utility as a function of action *a* for a negative exponential performance function and linear cost and benefit functions. Solid line: expectation. Dashed lines: Q25 and Q75. Middle panel: uncertainty levels (standard deviations) as indicated in the text. Left panel: uncertainties divided by 1.5. Right panel: uncertainties multiplied by 1.5

Chapter 13
Implementation of BDT Using Bayesian Networks

This chapter provides details on the implementation of BDT. As examples, we use similarly simple models as in Chap. 12, but now show explicitly how we extract information from them.

We present two different stochastic models that are consistent with the general graphical model, a fully linear and a partly nonlinear one. The first can be solved analytically, the second only numerically which we implement using the R-package `Nimble`.

We begin with the simplest form of graphical model. *Bayesian networks* (BN, also called *Bayesian Belief Networks* or BBN) are graphical models in the form of *directed acyclic graphs* (DAGs) whose edges are arrows and that do not allow any loops. The arrows indicate how a joint probability distribution can be decomposed into conditionally independent parts. We shall initially focus on *Gaussian Bayesian Networks* (GBNs).

A *GBN* is a multivariate Gaussian probability distribution depicted by a DAG. Every multivariate Gaussian is fully specified by its mean vector and covariance matrix but these are not shown in the DAG. Instead, the graph shows how the distribution can most efficiently be factorised. The following introduction to GBN is based on (Van Oijen, 2020, Chap. 15).

13.1   Three Ways to Specify a Multivariate Gaussian

The multivariate Gaussian underlying the GBN is fully specified by its mean vector and covariance matrix (or its inverse, the *precision matrix*). The diagonal of the

Supplementary Information The online version contains supplementary material available at https://doi.org/10.1007/978-3-031-16333-3_13

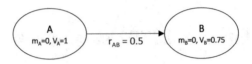

Fig. 13.1 DAG with means and conditional variances specified in the node-ellipses and edge labelled with the regression coefficient

covariance matrix gives the *unconditional variances* of the nodes, which quantify our uncertainty about the node-values when the values of the other nodes are not known yet.

Alternatively, we can quantify how much uncertainty we still have about each node after the values of all other nodes have become known. Those *conditional variances* together with the mean vector and the regression coefficients for each pair of nodes also constitute a full specification of the multivariate Gaussian underlying our GBN.

So, if we have a DAG for a GBN with n nodes and r edges, we can specify its multivariate Gaussian distribution in three ways:

1. $n \times 1$ mean vector + $n \times n$ covariance matrix,
2. $n \times 1$ mean vector + $n \times n$ precision matrix,
3. $n \times 1$ mean vector + $n \times 1$ vector of conditional variances + $r \times 1$ vector of regression coefficients.

Only the third method actually makes use of the information in the DAG, and it is also often the easiest to specify. The vector-information that it provides can be included in the DAG, which would make the graph fully self-explanatory. All we need to do for that is adding the mean and conditional variance to each node, and labelling each edge with the regression coefficient. See Fig. 13.1 for an example.

A convenient property of GBNs is that any two nodes for which the regression coefficient is zero are conditionally independent. That tells us that we do not need to draw an arrow between those nodes. On the other hand, GBNs are limited in that they can only represent linear relationships whose slopes are given by the regression coefficients R_{ij}. The strengths of the relationships can be assessed by inspecting the covariance matrix. Some nodes may be so closely correlated that the relationship is effectively a deterministic linear function.

13.1.1 Switching Between the Three Different Specifications of the Multivariate Gaussian

We can always switch between the three ways of specifying the multivariate Gaussian that we listed above. Conversion between specifications (1) and (2) is conceptually the easiest because the covariance and precision matrices are each

other's inverse. The conversion from (3) to (2) can be done using the algorithm
of Shachter and Kenley (1989), encoded in R as follows:

```
precMatrix <- function( nodes, Vcond, R ){
  n <- length(nodes) ; W <- 1 / Vcond[1]
  for(k in 2:n){
    rk       <- R[ k, 1:(k-1) ]
    W_top    <- cbind( W * Vcond[k] + rk %*% t(rk), -rk ) / Vcond[k]
    W_bottom <- cbind(                      -t(rk),   1 ) / Vcond[k]
    W        <- rbind( W_top, W_bottom ) }
  rownames(W) <- colnames(W) <- nodes
  return(W) }
```

This function has three arguments: `nodes`, `Vcond` and R. The first argument
is the vector of node-names. The second is an equally long vector of conditional
variances. And the third is a matrix R with zeroes everywhere except for the
elements R_{ij} that correspond to an edge from node j to node i in the DAG.

Castillo et al. (2008) provided an algorithm for the conversion from method (2)
to (3) that we implement here as follows:

```
VcondR <- function( W ) {
  n  <- dim(W)[1] ; Vcond <- rep( NA, n )
  Wk <- W         ; R     <- matrix( 0, nrow=n, ncol=n )
  for(k in n:2){
    ik       <- 1 : (k-1)
    Vcond[k] <- 1 / Wk[ k, k]
    R[k,ik]  <-    -Wk[ k,ik] * Vcond[k]
    Wk       <-    Wk[ik,ik] - as.matrix(R[k,ik]) %*% R[k,ik] / Vcond[k] }
  Vcond[1] <- 1 / Wk[1,1]
  return( list( Vcond=Vcond, R=zapsmall(R) ) ) }
```

13.2   Sampling from a GBN and Bayesian Updating

Because a GBN is a probability distribution, we can sample from it. This can be
done one node at a time, following the factorisation implied by the structure of the
DAG, but we can also do this using standard algorithms for sampling vectors from
the whole multivariate Gaussian in one go. The first method—which only involves
conditionally *univariate* Gaussians—will be computationally more efficient when
the network has many nodes because it avoids the inversion of the covariance matrix.

13.2.1　Updating a GBN When Information About Nodes Becomes Available

After we have specified our network, new information may become available. For example, the value of one or more nodes may become known through measurement. That information then affects the remaining nodes, so the whole network needs to be updated. In the case of GBNs, the 'posterior network' can be found analytically and we implement that analytical solution in R here. The algorithm operates on the covariance matrix of the GBN so for this task we need to provide the covariance specification of the GBN (method 1 in our list). Computationally more efficient ways that take advantage of the network structure take more steps and are not needed for the simple examples here.

Here is the code for the posterior mean and covariance matrix of a multivariate Gaussian distribution after we learn the values y for one or more of the nodes.

```
GaussCond <- function( mz, Sz, y ) {
  i <- 1 : ( length(mz) - length(y) )
  m  <- mz[i]   + Sz[i,-i] %*% solve(Sz[-i,-i]) %*% (y-mz[-i])
  S  <- Sz[i,i] - Sz[i,-i] %*% solve(Sz[-i,-i]) %*% Sz[-i,i]
  return( list( m=m, S=S ) ) }
```

In this code, the vector y (with length n_y) represents the nodes that become known, with the measurements corresponding to the last n_y values of the mean vector. The function returns the new mean vector and covariance matrix for the smaller network that remains when the known nodes are removed and the others updated.

We now have the machinery to carry out BDT using Bayesian Networks, as we show in the following example.

13.3　A Linear BDT Example Implemented as a GBN

In this section, we implement a simple linear example of BDT as a GBN. As always, we begin by drawing the DAG (Fig. 13.2). It shows that we see the utility as the difference between the benefit from forest growth (quantified as the yield class YC) and the cost from irrigation. Forest growth is increased by both rain and irrigation.

The distribution implied by Fig. 13.2 has the following mean vector μ, covariance matrix Σ and precision matrix W:

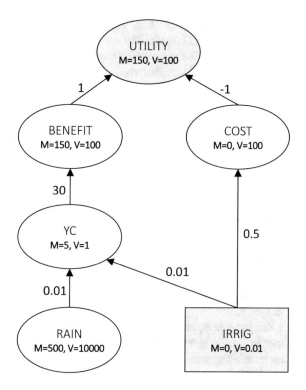

Fig. 13.2 Example of linear BDT represented by a DAG with six nodes and six edges. Each node shows the values of the prior mean and conditional variance. Each edge is labelled with the regression coefficient

Original network:

$$
\begin{bmatrix} RAIN \\ IRRIG \\ YC \\ BENEFIT \\ COST \\ UTILITY \end{bmatrix} : \quad \mu = \begin{bmatrix} 500 \\ 0 \\ 5 \\ 150 \\ 0 \\ 150 \end{bmatrix}; \quad \Sigma = \begin{bmatrix} 10000 & 0 & 100 & 3000 & 0 & 3000 \\ 0 & 0 & 0 & 0 & 0 & 0 \\ 100 & 0 & 2 & 60 & 0 & 60 \\ 3000 & 0 & 60 & 1900 & 0 & 1900 \\ 0 & 0 & 0 & 0 & 100 & -100 \\ 3000 & 0 & 60 & 1900 & -100 & 2100 \end{bmatrix};
$$

$$
W = \begin{bmatrix} 0 & 0 & -0.01 & 0 & 0 & 0 \\ 0 & 100 & -0.01 & 0 & 0 & 0 \\ -0.01 & -0.01 & 10 & -0.3 & 0 & 0 \\ 0 & 0 & -0.3 & 0.02 & -0.01 & -0.01 \\ 0 & 0 & 0 & -0.01 & 0.02 & 0.01 \\ 0 & 0 & 0 & -0.01 & 0.01 & 0.01 \end{bmatrix}.
$$

$$(13.1)$$

The covariance matrix shows that the *unconditional variance* of utility is 2100. This high value quantifies our uncertainty about utility when no information has been collected about any of the parent nodes, and therefore it is much higher than the *conditional variance* of utility which we had set at 100 (as indicated in Fig. 13.2).

We now update the network with an observed value for rain of 600 mm y^{-1}. That gives us the following mean vector and covariance matrix for the five remaining nodes:

Posterior network after accounting for RAIN:

$$
\begin{bmatrix} IRRIG \\ YC \\ BENEFIT \\ COST \\ UTILITY \end{bmatrix} : \quad \mu = \begin{bmatrix} 0 \\ 6 \\ 180 \\ 0 \\ 180 \end{bmatrix} ; \quad \Sigma = \begin{bmatrix} 0.01 & 0 & 0 & 0 & 0 \\ 0 & 1 & 30 & 0 & 30 \\ 0 & 30 & 1000 & 0 & 1000 \\ 0 & 0 & 0 & 100 & -100 \\ 0 & 30 & 1000 & -100 & 1200 \end{bmatrix} .
$$
$$(13.2)$$

We now want to update the network further with an 'observed' value for irrigation of 400 mm y^{-1}. We can do that in two equivalent ways. First, by starting from the original 6-node network and providing the information about both RAIN and IRRIG together. Secondly, by starting from the 5-node network that we have after providing a value for RAIN, and just providing the value for IRRIG. Adding the information about irrigation gives us the following mean vector and covariance matrix for the four remaining nodes:

Posterior network after accounting for RAIN and IRRIG:

$$
\begin{bmatrix} YC \\ BENEFIT \\ COST \\ UTILITY \end{bmatrix} : \quad \mu = \begin{bmatrix} 10 \\ 300 \\ 200 \\ 100 \end{bmatrix} ; \quad \Sigma = \begin{bmatrix} 1 & 30 & 0 & 30 \\ 30 & 1000 & 0 & 1000 \\ 0 & 0 & 100 & -100 \\ 30 & 1000 & -100 & 1200 \end{bmatrix} .
$$
$$(13.3)$$

The marginal distribution for utility changed considerably by adding the information about rain and then irrigation. The prior expectation for utility $E[U]$ was 150 (with variance V = 2100), after supplying the information on rain $E[U|rain = 600] = 180$ (V = 1200) and after setting irrigation at 400 mm y^{-1} we finally arrived at $E[U|rain = 600, irrig = 400] = 100$ (V = 1200). So the variance decreased strongly when we provided information about rain, but not when we added information about irrigation because that had low initial variance to begin with.

13.4 A Linear BDT Example Implemented Using `Nimble`

We continue with the same GM but this time implement it using R-package `Nimble`. This is intended to serve as an introduction to the use of numerical methods such as MCMC for BDT.

```
BDT.Code <- nimbleCode({
   RAIN      ~ dnorm( 500, sd= 100   )
   IRRIG     ~ dnorm(   0, sd=   0.1 )
   YC        <- (RAIN + IRRIG) * 0.01 + eps.YC
   BENEFIT <-   YC           * 30   + eps.BE
   COST      <-   IRRIG        * 0.5 + eps.CO
   UTILITY <-   BENEFIT - COST      + eps.UT
   eps.YC    ~ dnorm( 0, sd= 1 )
   eps.BE    ~ dnorm( 0, sd=10 )
   eps.CO    ~ dnorm( 0, sd=10 )
   eps.UT    ~ dnorm( 0, sd=10 )
} )
```

As before, we shall sample from the prior distribution for utility and two posterior distributions conditional on data for rain and irrigation. However, this time the posterior distributions are not found analytically but simulated using MCMC. Apart from this numerical approach, the implementation of the GM using `Nimble` is equivalent to the GBN above.

We run the MCMCs and show prior and posterior samples of utility in Fig. 13.3. As expected, the means and variances are very close to the values that we found analytically from the GBN in the previous section.

13.4.1 Varying IRRIG to Identify the Value for Which E[U] Is Maximized

For a proper application of BDT, we need to vary the control nodes (here just 'IRRIG') continuously along their domain to identify the value for which the expectation of the utility $E[U]$ is maximal. We set RAIN at 600 mm y^{-1} and vary IRRIG from 0 to 500 mm y^{-1} in steps of 100 mm y^{-1}.

The results are shown in Fig. 13.4. In this linear example, $E[U]$ varies linearly with irrigation and the optimum is found at IRRIG = 0. Of course, this result is quite trivial because the costs of 1 mm of irrigation were set at 0.5 whereas 1 mm of irrigation gave only 0.01 unit of extra growth at a benefit per unit growth of 30, so benefits per mm irrigation were only 0.3. Irrigation costs thus always exceed benefits and the optimum is zero.

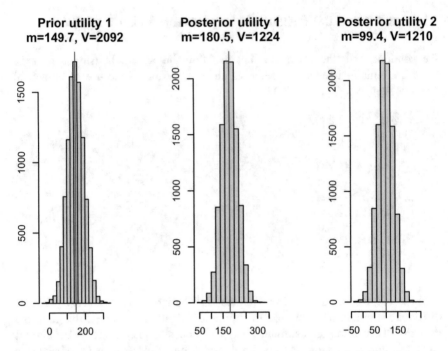

Fig. 13.3 Linear model. Sampling from the marginal Gaussian distribution for utility using the R-package Nimble. Left: prior. Middle: posterior after setting rain at 600 mm y^{-1}. Right: posterior after additionally setting irrigation at 400 mm y^{-1}

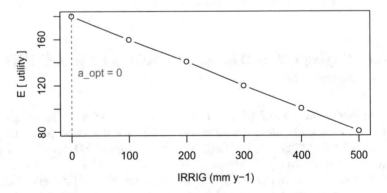

Fig. 13.4 BDT for a linear network: identifying the level of irrigation for which the expectation of utility is maximized

13.5   A Nonlinear BDT Example Implemented Using `Nimble`

We now make the decision problem more interesting by making the dependence of
YC on water supply (= rain + irrigation) nonlinear. We do this by changing a single
line in the `Nimble`-code:

```
YC <- 50 * (1-exp(-0.001*(RAIN + IRRIG))) + eps.YC
```

Despite this change, we are still working with the graphical model of Fig. 13.2
as far as the nodes and arrows are concerned. But the model is not a GBN anymore,
and the dependence of YC on RAIN and IRRIG can no longer be fully specified
with a regression coefficient.

We begin by running the same three MCMCs as before in the linear example.
Samples from the resulting utility distributions are shown in Fig. 13.5.

And we also carry out the Bayesian decision analysis as before, but this time
we need to inspect a wider range of irrigation levels, as we can see in Fig. 13.6.
$E[U]$ now no longer varies linearly with irrigation, and an optimum is found around
$500\,\text{mm}\ y^{-1}$.

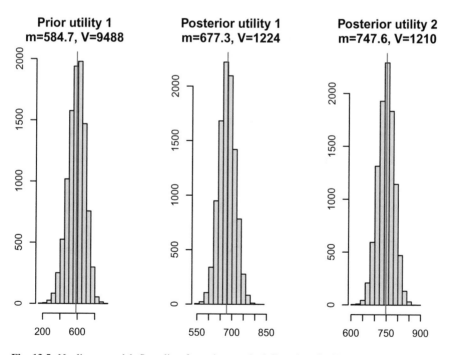

Fig. 13.5 Nonlinear model. Sampling from the marginal Gaussian distribution for utility using
the R-package `Nimble`. Left: prior. Middle: posterior after setting rain at $600\,\text{mm}\ y^{-1}$. Right:
posterior after additionally setting irrigation at $400\,\text{mm}\ y^{-1}$

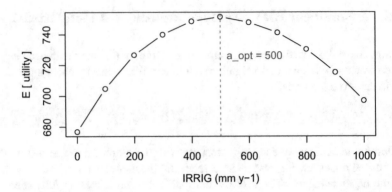

Fig. 13.6 BDT for a nonlinear network: identifying the level of irrigation for which the expectation of utility is maximized

Chapter 14
A Spatial Example: Forestry in Scotland

The main purpose of this example is to show how theory developed in earlier chapters can be applied to a spatial decision problem where model inputs and outputs are maps of a geographical region. We also intend this and the following chapters to be a repository of succinct and efficient R-algorithms for spatial problems in PRA and BDT.

We begin by presenting the data for Scotland used here. Then we introduce the forest productivity function, and show how to derive a so-called *Gaussian Process (GP) emulator* for it. As will be explained in more detail below, such emulators are stochastic approximations of deterministic models that are used to accelerate computation. We apply the original function and the emulator to the Scottish data, showing that they produce similar but not identical results. In the next chapter, we use these tools in a simple binary BDT-problem where benefits from forest productivity are offset by costs of irrigation.

14.1 A Decision Problem: Forest Irrigation in Scotland

We shall be examining algorithms for PRA and BDT in this chapter. This will mostly be done using a single example: deciding where to irrigate forests in Scotland. We show how we processed publicly available WorldClim data on precipitation to create R data structures called *RasterStacks* containing time series of precipitation for grid cells of width 2.5 minutes that cover Scotland. These data structures allow for efficient parallel computation of PRA and BDT for all cells. Our example will not be realistic in that we shall ignore some parameter uncertainties and

Supplementary Information The online version contains supplementary material available at https://doi.org/10.1007/978-3-031-16333-3_14

M. van Oijen, M. Brewer, *Probabilistic Risk Analysis and Bayesian Decision Theory*, SpringerBriefs in Statistics, https://doi.org/10.1007/978-3-031-16333-3_14

forest productivity will be calculated as a simple function of water availability (precipitation and irrigation) and altitude. A more realistic example would follow the same methodology but be slower to calculate.

14.2 Computational Demand of BDT and Emulation

The computational demand of BDT can be high. As mentioned before, there are four main reasons for this:

1. Double iteration: over parameter uncertainty and over action choice.
2. Complexity of the Bayesian Hierarchical Model (BHM) as represented by our graphical model (GM) for the decision problem.
3. Complexity and slowness of any process-based models (PBMs) used.
4. Repetition of the action optimisation over time and space, as will usually be required since most environmental problems are spatio-temporal.

An increasingly common method of reducing computational demand is to replace part of the calculations by emulation. We can, for example, replace a slow PBM with an emulator that predicts the PBM-output for any choice of input values, without running the PBM itself. Because this introduces uncertainty about the quality of the output estimation, stochastic emulators are generally used that provide a measure of uncertainty with each prediction. Gaussian Process (GP) emulators tend to be the default choice. In our application of BDT to forest planting, emulation can be applied at various stages. We can:

- use emulators in our GM for the PBMs to emulate *forest yield* prediction as a function of x and θ,
- use emulators in our GM for *utility* itself as a function of a, x and θ,
- or even one step further: use emulators for the *expectation of utility*,
- or emulating the ultimate goal: the optimal action *a.opt*.

We include an example of forest yield emulation by GP in this chapter. As noted above, our central problem of Scottish forestry calculates forest productivity as a simple function of water availability and altitude instead of using a complex PBM. This does not affect the algorithms for deriving and applying the emulator while speeding up their execution.

14.3 Data

We began by using the R-package `raster` to download information about the spatial extent of Great Britain from the GADM database. We cropped this to Scotland.

```
spdf_GBR <- getData( 'GADM', country="GBR", level=0, path="data" ) # GB
spdf_SCO <- crop   ( spdf_GBR, extent(-7.7,-1.8,54.5,58.6) ) # Scotland
ext_SCO  <- extent ( spdf_SCO )
```

The next step was to download precipitation data for Scotland. WorldClim (https://www.worldclim.org/data/index.html) provides monthly data for both *climate* (30-year averages) and *weather* (2000–2018). The data is cumbersome: one has to begin by downloading high-spatial resolution data for the whole globe, then crop these to the regions of interest before storing the cropped files locally. However, WorldClim data are useful in that they are freely available, comprehensive (the climate data cover the five weather variables used by many process-based models: radiation, temperature, atmospheric vapour pressure, wind speed, precipitation) and are of apparently high quality without any gaps or ourliers.

WorldClim's climatic data are for all five variables whereas WorldClim's weather data are just for temperature and rainfall. The weather data are at lower spatial resolution (2.5 minutes) than the climate data (30 seconds).

We downloaded monthly precipitation data from WorldClim as tif-files. The identifiers `dir_WC_prec.2000_2009` and `dir_WC_prec.2010_2018` in the next code chunk refer to local directories where the tif-files were stored. Subsequent code lines show how we cropped the areal coverage to Scotland (Fig. 14.1), and aggregated the data to 19 annual precipitation maps for the years 2000–2018. The maps were stored in R data structures called RasterStacks (see https://www.benjaminbell.co.uk/2018/02/rasterstacks-and-rasterplot.html), which allow for easy parallel post-processing.

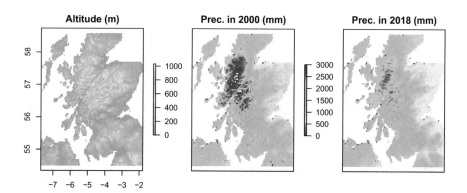

Fig. 14.1 Scotland: altitude and precipitation in 2000 and 2018

```
s_prec.mon                <- stack( c(
  list.files( dir_WC_prec.2000_2009, ".tif", full.names=T ),
  list.files( dir_WC_prec.2010_2018, ".tif", full.names=T ) ) )
s_prec.mon                <- crop(s_prec.mon, ext_SCO)
s_prec.mon                <- s_prec.mon[[1:228]] # Keep Jan 2000 to Dec 2018
names(s_prec.mon)         <- str_sub( names(s_prec.mon), -7, -1 )
years                     <- rep( 2000:2018, each=12 )
s_prec                    <- stackApply( s_prec.mon, years, fun=sum )
```

In like manner, we downloaded and cropped data on altitude:

```
r_alt_WesternEurope    <- getData( 'worldclim', var='alt', res=0.5,
                                   lon=-4.75, lat= 56.55 )
r_alt_highres          <- crop( r_alt_WesternEurope, ext_SCO )
r_alt                  <- resample( r_alt_highres, s_prec )
```

Figure 14.1 shows the altitude map of Scotland and examples of annual precipitation (years 2000 and 2018).

14.4   A Simple Model for Forest Yield Class (YC)

In this section, we define a simple nonlinear model for the yield class of wood production (YC; $m^3\,ha^{-1}\,y^{-1}$) and apply it to data for Scotland. We assume that YC is a negative exponential function of rainfall (R) and a linear function of altitude (A):

$$YC = 10 * (1 - exp(-R/1000)) * (1 - A/1000)$$

We embed this model in an R-function as follows:

```
YC <- function( x ) {
  alt <- x[1]  ; prec <- x[2]
  YC  <- max(0, 10 * (1-exp(-prec/1000)) * (1-alt/1000) )
  return( YC ) }
```

To show this function in action, we (1) select the precipitation data for 2000 from the RasterStack and (2) calculate YC for all grid cells. Both steps can be carried out with short code from the R-package `raster`:

```
r_prec_2000 <- raster ( s_prec, layer=1 )
r_YC        <- overlay( r_alt, r_prec_2000, fun=YC )
```

The YC-values for 2000 that we calculated in this way are shown in the top left panel of Fig. 14.2.

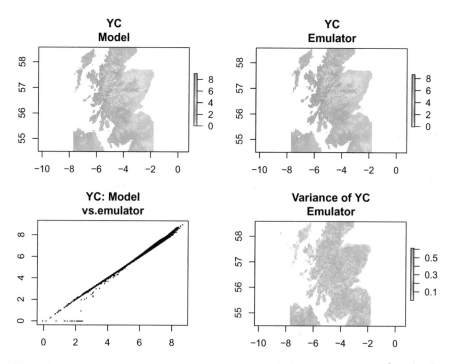

Fig. 14.2 Top left: outputs from the original nonlinear model for yield class (YC, $m^3\,ha^{-1}\,y^{-1}$) applied to precipitation data from the year 2000. Top right: emulated YC. Bottom left: original outputs vs. emulated values. Bottom right: emulator uncertainty (kriging variance)

14.5   Emulation

In this section, we derive an emulator for the YC-model and apply the emulator to the altitude and weather data for Scotland. We then check whether the emulator gives similar values as the original model.

To prepare for model emulation, we need to select a small number of points, so-called 'design points,' for which we know the values of the inputs as well as the outputs calculated with the original model. Here we sample from uniform distributions for altitude and precipitation but more sophisticated designs (such as Latin Hypercube sampling) can be chosen.

```
n_design    <- 50
alt_design  <- runif( n_design, 0, 1000 )
prec_design <- runif( n_design, 0, 3000 )
YC_design   <- sapply( 1:n_design, function(i) {
  YC( c(alt_design[i],prec_design[i]) ) } )
```

We shall be deriving a GP-emulator such that the emulator produces exactly the same productivity values as the original model when the input-vector is a design

point, while elsewhere differences and uncertainties increase with distance. The
degree to which proximity confers similarity is captured by parameters: correlation
length and asymptotic variance. In our simple example here, we assume that these
parameters are known (which makes our approach akin to geostatistical techniques
such as classical *kriging* where these parameters would be estimated from the same
data but subsequently treated as known quantities), but when applying emulation to
a realistic example these parameters should be estimated with quantified uncertainty.
This can be done by means of *Bayesian kriging* (Van Oijen, 2020, Chap. 22).

```
x1 <- alt_design   ; x2 <- prec_design       ; y <- YC_design
ny <- length(y)
Vy <- 1            ; phi <- 1000
x  <- cbind(x1,x2) ; dx  <- as.matrix( dist(x) ) ; Sy <- exp( -dx/phi ) * Vy
```

Using the design points, we derive the emulator. With known emulator variance
and correlation length, this can be done analytically with the following code (taken
from Van Oijen, 2020, Chap. 14):

```
GP.est <- function( x, y, Sy, mb, Sb, X=cbind(1,x) ) {
  Sb_y <- solve( solve(Sb) + t(X) %*% solve(Sy) %*% X )
  mb_y <- Sb_y %*% ( solve(Sb) %*% mb + t(X) %*% solve(Sy) %*% y )
  return( list( "mb_y"=mb_y, "Sb_y"=Sb_y ) ) }


mb   <- c(0,0,0) ; Sb <- diag(1,3) ; X <- cbind(1,x)
b_y  <- GP.est( x, y, Sy, mb=mb, Sb=Sb, X=X )
mb_y <- b_y$mb_y; Sb_y <- b_y$Sb_y
```

14.6   Application of the Emulator

Convenient code for using the GP-emulator in prediction was presented by Van
Oijen (2020, Chap. 14):

```
GP.pred <- function(x0,x,y,Sy,phi,mb_y,Sb_y,X0=c(1,x0),X=cbind(1,x)) {
  dx0  <- if( is.vector(x) ) { abs(x-x0)
          } else { sapply(1:length(y),function(i){dist(rbind(x0,x[i,]))}) }
  C0   <- Sy[1] * exp( -dx0/phi )
  m0_y <- X0 %*% mb_y - t(C0) %*% solve(Sy) %*% (X %*% mb_y - y)
    a <- X0 - t(C0) %*% solve(Sy) %*% X
  S0_y <- Sy[1] - t(C0) %*% solve(Sy) %*% C0 + a %*% Sb_y %*% t(a)
  return( list( "m0_y"=m0_y, "S0_y"=S0_y ) ) }


x0   <- c(0,0) ; X0 <- c(1,x0)
y0_y <- GP.pred( x0, x, y, Sy, phi, mb_y, Sb_y, X0=X0, X=X )
m0_y <- y0_y$m0_y ; S0_y <- y0_y$S0_y
```

We make the emulator easily accessible by embedding it in two R-functions
YC_em and YC_em.S:

```
YC_em <- function( x0 ) {
  YC <- GP.pred( x0, x, y, Sy, phi, mb_y, Sb_y,
                 X0=c(1,x0), X=cbind(1,x) )$m0_y
  return( YC ) }
YC_em.S <- function( x0 ) {
  S  <- GP.pred( x0, x, y, Sy, phi, mb_y, Sb_y,
                 X0=c(1,x0), X=cbind(1,x) )$S0_y
  return( S ) }
```

Because the emulator is stochastic, we defined two functions. The first function
produces the predictive mean and the second one the predictive variance (or 'kriging
variance').

So at this point we can choose the original function YC() or the emulator
YC_em() to predict forest productivity. This time we choose the emulator and
apply it to the altitude and rainfall data for Scotland, using R's raster-package
functionality. As before, we use the year 2000 as the example:

```
r_YC_em   <- overlay( r_alt, r_prec_2000, fun=YC_em   )
r_YC_em.S <- overlay( r_alt, r_prec_2000, fun=YC_em.S )
```

The results from using the emulator are shown in Fig. 14.2 together with the YC
as calculated by the original model. Clearly, the results are very similar indicating
that either method can be chosen. However, emulation does incur the cost of some
uncertainty in estimation which is shown in the bottom-right panel of the same
figure.

Chapter 15
Spatial BDT Using Model and Emulator

We now use the model and emulator in our BDT problem concerning forestry in
Scotland. We want to decide where we should irrigate and where not. So our choice
of action a is a matter of setting the level of irrigation, which we denote as $IRRIG$.
To keep this example simple, we allow only two action levels: $IRRIG = 0$
vs. $IRRIG = 500\,$mm.

We ignore (for now) all parameter and input uncertainties.

We already showed $E[z|a = 0]$ in Fig. 14.2, where z=YC and where a=0 refers
to the absence of irrigation ($IRRIG = 0$). To calculate the benefits associated with
forest production, we need to multiply z with money received per unit of z (YC).
We assume that the wood price is a constant $ky = 30$. In this case, without any
irrigation costs, *utility* is simply these expected benefits, so here $E[U|a = 0] =
E[ky * z|a = 0]$. Because we are ignoring uncertainties, these expectations are
deterministic functions of precipitation and altitude.

We carry out the calculations both with the original model and the emulator.

```
ky <- 30 ;    r_U <- r_YC * ky ;    r_U_em <- r_YC_em * ky
```

Next, we repeat the calculations but with irrigation. To calculate the utility
associated with that action choice, we need to consider not just the benefits but

Supplementary Information The online version contains supplementary material available at
https://doi.org/10.1007/978-3-031-16333-3_15

85
M. van Oijen, M. Brewer, *Probabilistic Risk Analysis and Bayesian
Decision Theory*, SpringerBriefs in Statistics,
https://doi.org/10.1007/978-3-031-16333-3_15

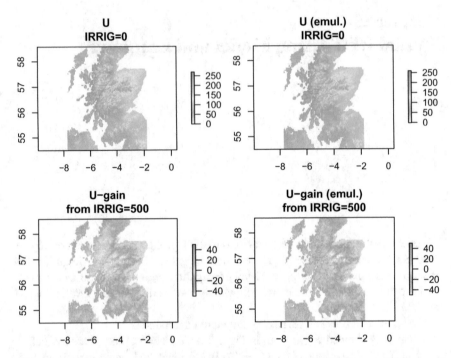

Fig. 15.1 Top: utility in the year 2000 without irrigation. Bottom: gain in utility with irrigation of 500 mm y^{-1}. Left: original model. Right: emulator

also the costs of irrigation. We assume that the costs per mm irrigation are constant: $ka = 0.1$.

```
IRRIG          <- 500
r_YC.IRRIG     <- overlay( r_alt, r_prec_2000 + IRRIG, fun=YC    )
r_YC_em.IRRIG  <- overlay( r_alt, r_prec_2000 + IRRIG, fun=YC_em )


ka             <- 0.1
r_U.IRRIG      <- r_YC.IRRIG    * ky - IRRIG * ka
r_U_em.IRRIG   <- r_YC_em.IRRIG * ky - IRRIG * ka
```

The results of the utility calculations are shown in Fig. 15.1. The figure shows that irrigation only leads to utility-gain in some drier eastern coastal regions of Scotland.

In this example, the decision problem is simple. Because there are only two possible actions (zero or 500 mm y^{-1} irrigation), whichever of the two leads to the highest expected utility is the optimal action to be selected. And because we ignored uncertainties, finding locations where irrigation is advisable simplifies to inspecting the map of utility-gain due to irrigation and selecting those locations where the gain is positive, i.e. some eastern locations.

Some differences between the original model and the emulator are visible in the high-rainfall Western Highlands of Scotland, where only the emulator suggests that irrigation approaches positive utility-gain. This shows that emulators are especially unreliable under extreme conditions where kriging variance is high (Fig. 14.2). In the remainder of this book, we shall only be using the original model.

15.1 Multiple Action Levels

We now repeat the spatial BDT problem, but this time allow for more action levels than just two. Our purpose here is to show that this can also be implemented very easily using R's `raster` package.

```
nI     <- 10 ;   layers <- 1:nI ;   IRRIG <- (layers-1)*50
s_U.a <- raster(ext_SCO)
for(i in layers) {
  r_YC.a <- overlay( r_alt, r_prec_2000 + IRRIG[i], fun=YC )
  r_U.a  <- r_YC.a * ky - IRRIG[i] * ka
  s_U.a  <- addLayer( s_U.a, r_U.a ) }

layer.max <- function(x, ...){
  max_idx <- which.max(x)   # Get the max
  ifelse(length(max_idx)==0,return(NA),return(max_idx)) }
layer.amax <- calc( s_U.a, layer.max )
a.opt      <- (layer.amax-1)*50
```

Figure 15.2 shows the outcome from this decision problem.

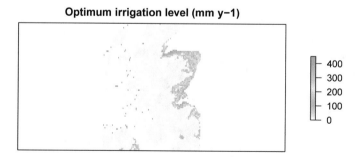

Optimum irrigation level (mm y−1)

400
300
200
100
0

Fig. 15.2 Outcome from a decision problem where action choice was between a large number of irrigation levels

Chapter 16
Linkages Between PRA and BDT

In this chapter, we discuss the relationship between PRA, as developed in this book, and BDT. We show that the latter's maximisation of utility-expectation (BDT) equates to minimising a 'corrected' form of risk. For discussion of the linkages between older (discrete and less comprehensively probabilistic) forms of PRA and BDT, see Borgonovo et al. (2018).

We begin by carrying out a PRA with utility u as the system variable, using the same negative exponential example that we used for BDT in Chap. 14. The idea is to compare PRA and BDT—how much can one learn from the two approaches?

The first step in PRA is to define the system variable (here u) and the environment variable which we in previous chapters denoted as x. But is the x that we specified for the BDT example also the appropriate environment variable for PRA? When we inspect our negative exponential performance function fy(), we see that it defines an asymptotic dependence on $x + a$, so that sum is a better choice for our environment variable. Note that it is the sum of an exogenous variable x (e.g. rain) and an action variable a that is under human control (e.g. irrigation). As threshold value, we choose $thr = 0$.

Increasing the action a will decrease the frequency with which the environment variable will drop below the threshold. In other words, this is an example of an action that will decrease $p[H]$ but may have little impact on V. R will then primarily be reduced because of the effect of the action a on $p[H]$ rather than on V.

[Note that if we would have chosen x as the environment variable in our PRA (instead of $x + a$), then increasing a would leave $p[H]$ unaffected but reduce V. There is nothing fundamentally wrong with that approach, but the interpretation where a is part of the environment variable 'water availability' seems more natural.]

Supplementary Information The online version contains supplementary material available at https://doi.org/10.1007/978-3-031-16333-3_16

M. van Oijen, M. Brewer, *Probabilistic Risk Analysis and Bayesian Decision Theory*, SpringerBriefs in Statistics, https://doi.org/10.1007/978-3-031-16333-3_16

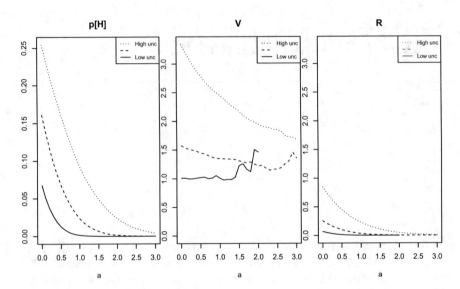

Fig. 16.1 PRAs on data generated for BDT

We run the PRA for all values of the action a that we examined in the BDT, and we again compare results for different levels of uncertainty. We use the code for PRA that we developed in Chap. 4. The results shown in Fig. 16.1 partly confirm our expectations. We see that $p[H]$ indeed changes the most when varying a, but V also changes, especially in the high-uncertainty scenario. The figure further shows that when $p[H]$ becomes close to zero, it becomes difficult to estimate V because of small sampling size for estimating $E[z|H]$.

16.1   Risk Management

The PRAs that we just carried out for our BDT-example show that we can make risks as small as we want by increasing the action a. But remember that the risk is the *difference* between two expectations for the system variable of interest (here the utility u), and both expectations include the same cost of the action. In other words, increasing a may reduce R to zero but that may not be desirable because the action costs $ka \times a$ will increase and thereby decrease u itself. Another way of looking at this is that a mitigating action may make a hazard factor (here x) irrelevant and thus stabilise system performance at the cost of reducing utility even in years when the hazard factor would not have been a problem anyway [Note that this is exactly how paying for insurance works.].

16.2   The Relationship Between Utility Maximisation in BDT and Risk Assessment in PRA: R_c

Let's examine the relationship between risk R and utility u, still using the same example. Because u is our system variable of interest, R is defined as:

$$R = E[u|\neg H] - E[u]. \tag{16.1}$$

So maximising $E[u]$ is the same as minimising $R - E[u|\neg H]$. We interpret the latter as 'risk corrected for costs and benefits' and denote it as R_c:

$$\begin{aligned} R_c &= R - E[u|\neg H] \\ &= R + E[ka|\neg H] \times a - E[ky \times y|\neg H]. \end{aligned} \tag{16.2}$$

So BDT can be formulated equally as maximising expected utility $E[u]$ or minimising corrected risk R_c.

Let's now verify that the corrected risk is indeed minimised at the same values of the action a that maximise expected utility. Figure 16.2 shows the results for the same three levels of uncertainty that we explored above, and we see that the smallest values of R_c are indeed found for the same values of a as maximising $E[u]$ did before (Fig. 12.3).

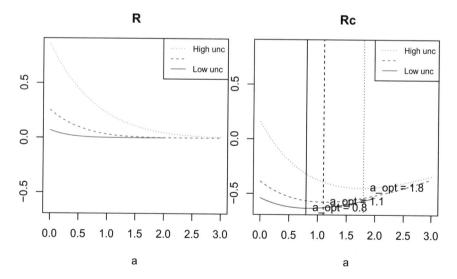

Fig. 16.2 Impact of action a on risk calculated from data generated for BDT. Left: uncorrected risk R, always decreasing with increasing a. Right: corrected risk R_c, reaching an uncertainty-dependent minimum at finite a

Of course R_c cannot be written as the product of $p[H]$ and V, so it does not replace R which can be decomposed. Our intention in defining R_c was solely to clarify the relationship between risk and utility.

16.3   Simplified Accounting for Both Benefits and Costs of the Action: R_b

Our definition of R_c (Eq. (16.2)), which makes it identical to $-E[u]$, involves *conditional* expectations for ka, ky and y for the *non-hazardous* domain of $x + a$. However, the effect of the action a on those variables might be quite similar in the hazardous domain. Let's now define R_b as the risk only corrected using unconditional expectations:

$$R_b = R + E[ka] \times a - E[ky] \times E[y]. \tag{16.3}$$

Note that the last term (product of expectations) implies that we ignore any possible correlation between ky and y, but that will generally be a plausible assumption anyway. If we calculate R_b for different values of a, we get the results of Fig. 16.3. We see that these show different optimal values of a than what we found when using R_c (or $E[u]$) but overall the results are similar. So sometimes the use of R_b may be good enough.

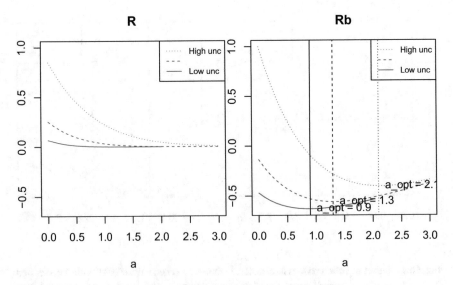

Fig. 16.3 Cost- and benefit-adjusted risk R_b using data generated for BDT

16.4 Only Correcting for Costs: R_a

If an action a only affected $p[H]$ while leaving $y|\neg H$ unchanged, then we could simplify our definition of a corrected risk by only accounting for the *costs* of a and not its benefits for y. We define such a simple 'cost-corrected R' as follows:

$$R_a = R + E[ka] \times a. \tag{16.4}$$

Note that we correct R for the *expectation* of costs because we treat the specific costs ka as an uncertain variable to which we assign a probability distribution rather than a known constant.

In the present example, we would not expect an analysis of the response of R_a to varying a to be useful, because clearly a does have an effect on benefits here. But let's do so anyway—we show the results in Fig. 16.4.

We see that R_a is minimised at lower values of a than R_c and R_b were because we are ignoring the beneficial effects of a on y. However, we still see that increasing uncertainty warrants choosing higher values of a. We conclude that there may be cases where it is useful to calculate R_a especially when the action a predominantly affects $p[H]$ and nothing else.

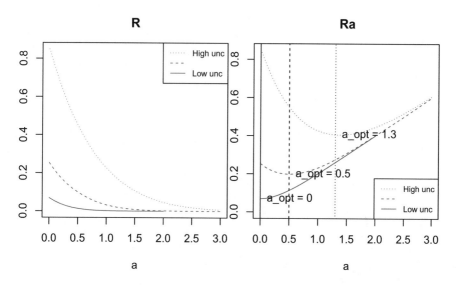

Fig. 16.4 Cost-adjusted risk R_a using data generated for BDT

Chapter 17
PRA vs. BDT in the Spatial Example

In this chapter, we examine the relationship between Bayesian decision theory (BDT) and probabilistic risk analysis (PRA) more closely. Our YC-model is the same as in the previously introduced spatial example, and our aim is also the same: we want to decide whether we should irrigate or not. But this time we base our decision not on a single year but on the whole time series of 19 years. The time series for each grid cell tells us, probabilistically, what level of precipitation we can expect there. The choice for each grid cell is then between irrigating and not irrigating. We shall decide to use irrigation in those locations where it increases the expectation for utility $E[U]$, calculated from the 19 years of data. We aim to show that locations where irrigation increases $E[U]$ are also the locations where it decreases the *corrected risk* R_c that we defined in Chap. 16.

We begin by calculating forest productivity for each of the 19 years, and store the productivities in RasterStacks:

```
s_YC   <- s_YC.IRRIG <- setValues( s_prec, NA )
IRRIG <- 500
for( y in 1:19 ) {
  r_prec.y      <- raster    ( s_prec, layer=y )
  r_YC.y        <- overlay   ( r_alt, r_prec.y           , fun=YC )
  r_YC.IRRIG.y  <- overlay   ( r_alt, r_prec.y + IRRIG, fun=YC )
  s_YC          <- setValues( s_YC       , getValues(r_YC.y       ), layer=y )
  s_YC.IRRIG    <- setValues( s_YC.IRRIG, getValues(r_YC.IRRIG.y), layer=y )
}
```

Supplementary Information The online version contains supplementary material available at https://doi.org/10.1007/978-3-031-16333-3_17

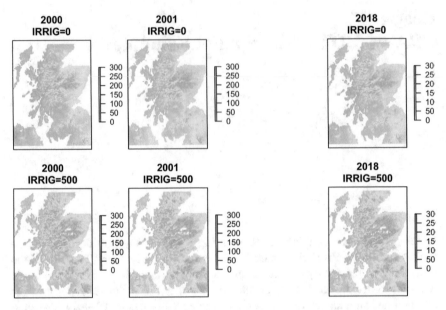

Fig. 17.1 Utility in 2000, 2001 and 2018. Top row: no irrigation. Bottom row: irrigation at 500 mm y^{-1}

Calculating utility-maps for each of the 19 years is then straightforward:

```
ky <- 30 ; ka <- 0.1
s_U       <- s_YC       * ky
s_U.IRRIG <- s_YC.IRRIG * ky - IRRIG * ka
```

Figure 17.1 shows utility maps for three of the 19 years, for conditions with and without irrigation.

Figure 17.2 shows $E[U]$, i.e. the mean values of utility over the 19 years.

When applying PRA to a sample of observations, we may face the problem that the observations are all in the hazardous domain or all in the non-hazardous domain. In such cases we lack information about the expectation value for the z variable in the non-observed domain. However, to maintain consistency in the calculations of risk R and the *corrected risk*, i.e. $R_c = R - E[z|\neg H] = -E[z]$, we define the unobservable expectations as $E[z|H] = min(z)$ (in case $p[H] = 0$) and $E[z|\neg H] = max(z)$ (in case $p[H] = 1$). This is equivalent to carrying out the PRA and R_c calculation in the limit of the hazardous threshold approaching $min(x)$ resp. $max(x)$ for a non-decreasing function $z(x)$.

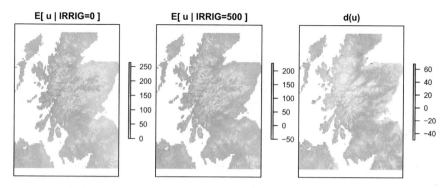

Fig. 17.2 Mean utility. Left: no irrigation. Middle: irrigation = 500 mm y^{-1}. Right: utility-gain from irrigation

We modify the earlier defined PRA-function accordingly. As intended, our new version of the function provides estimates of $p[H]$, V and R even when none or all of the x-values are in the hazardous domain.

```
    Ez_H <- mean( z[H] ) ; Ez_notH <- mean( z[-H] )
    }
    pH <- nH / n ; V <- Ez_notH - Ez_H ; R <- Ez_notH - Ez
    return( c( pH=pH, V=V, R=R,
                Ez=Ez, Ez_H=Ez_H, Ez_notH=Ez_notH ) ) }
```

An alternative approach would be to move to a distribution-based approach, e.g. by fitting a Gaussian or extreme value distribution to the x-data. We can then always generate a large enough sample from that distribution such that x-values from both the hazardous and the non-hazardous domains are included.

Figure 17.3 shows probabilistic risk analyses (PRA) for utility, based on each cell's 19-year time series of water availability with a hazardous threshold of 1500 mm y^{-1}. Note that there is a separate PRA for each cell, so the maps summarise results from a very large number of PRAs carried out in parallel.

Figure 17.4 shows the corrected risk for utility, defined as $R - E[z|\neg H]$.

The results confirm that maximising $E[U]$ (Fig. 17.2) gives exactly the same results as minimising R_c (Fig. 17.4).

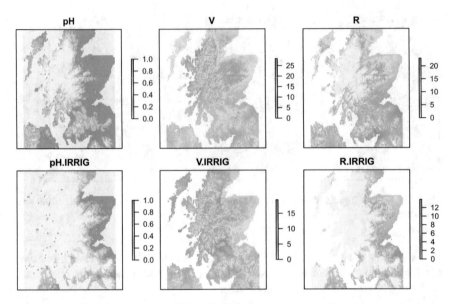

Fig. 17.3 PRA based on data for 2000–2018. Top row: no irrigation. Bottom row: irrigation = 500 mm y^{-1}

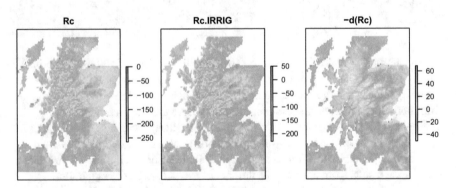

Fig. 17.4 Corrected risk for utility. Left: no irrigation. Middle: irrigation as above. Right: decrease in corrected risk due to irrigation

Chapter 18
Three-Component PRA in the Spatial Example

We shall not show any details of a 3-component PRA here—there are no special problems—but just point out that R's `raster` package makes it easy to calculate a spatially aggregated map for *exposure*, defined as the fraction of an area that has experienced drought at least once in the observational record (see Chap. 11). This is equivalent to counting cells where $p[H] > 0$, so we define an exposure-function accordingly and apply it to the $p[H]$-raster:

```
exposure <- function( pH, ... ){
  pH <- pH[!is.na(pH)] ; n <- length(pH) ; nE <- length( pH[pH>0] )
  if(n>0)  { Q <- nE/n
    } else { Q <- NA }
  return( Q ) }

r_Q <- aggregate( r_pH, fact=4, fun=exposure )
```

Figure 18.1 is the exposure map of Scotland that shows for regions of 4×4 grid cells what fraction of the cells experienced at least one drought year in 2000–2018.

Supplementary Information The online version contains supplementary material available at https://doi.org/10.1007/978-3-031-16333-3_18

M. van Oijen, M. Brewer, *Probabilistic Risk Analysis and Bayesian Decision Theory*, SpringerBriefs in Statistics, https://doi.org/10.1007/978-3-031-16333-3_18

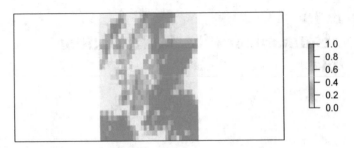

Fig. 18.1 Exposure to drought, calculated for regions of 4 × 4 grid cells

Chapter 19
Discussion

19.1 PRA and Its Application

This book has presented various forms of PRA. We started from the simplest form: sampling-based, single-category, single-threshold, two-component PRA. That was followed by alternatives or extensions for all those PRA-qualifiers. Mathematical equations and R-code were given for all the new types of PRA, as well as examples of their application to virtual data sets. We also presented equations and code for uncertainty quantification for risk and its components.

PRA as developed here, in all its forms, is based on the joint probability distribution $p[x, z]$ for an environmental variable x and a system variable z. Information about this distribution can come from measurement data or model output: the theory applies to both sources of information.

We started by defining hazardous conditions as x being below a certain threshold. We then extended this by allowing for multiple thresholds to subdivide the hazardous region into multiple intervals. In that way, the PRA can distinguish between different levels of hazard severity and quantify hazard probability and system vulnerability for each level.

In practical application there may also be a desire to subdivide the hazardous region not by intervals of one variable x, but by different categories of hazard, leading to 'categorical PRA.' This can be useful when different hazard variables are present, e.g. drought, flood, windthrow, infestation. Covariation of multiple hazard variables x_i is common (Hao et al., 2020; Venäläinen et al., 2020; Zscheischler et al., 2020), and copulas may be used in forming their joint distribution.

Another extension to PRA that we introduced was to decompose risk not in two but three components, by adding the component *exposure*. This can be useful in spatially distributed application of PRA where exposure is measured by the size of the area subject to the hazard.

M. van Oijen, M. Brewer, *Probabilistic Risk Analysis and Bayesian Decision Theory*, SpringerBriefs in Statistics, https://doi.org/10.1007/978-3-031-16333-3_19

The type of PRA to choose will vary between application domains. The optimal choice will depend on the nature of x and z, the main questions of interest, and the availability of measurement data and/or model output.

19.2   Data and Computational Demand of PRA

We distinguished three ways in which PRA can be implemented: sampling-, distribution- and model-based. Data needs will increase in that order because of the need to fit a probability distribution or a hierarchical model. Such distribution or model-fitting needs to be carried out with great care: the study of copulas and of extreme value theory (e.g. Butler et al. (2007) and Serinaldi et al. (2020)) has shown how sensitive any risk analysis is to the behaviour of tails of distributions, and how difficult they are to quantify when data availability is limited.

In the case of distribution-based PRA, there is a need to explore uncertainties associated with density estimation. We mentioned how semi-Bayesian information criteria such as AIC and BIC are used to select copulas, and fully Bayesian methods of distribution selection exist as well (e.g. Shen et al., 2013).

In the case of model-based PRA, it is generally unlikely that model error (also called 'discrepancy') is independent of x, so rich data sets are required to estimate variation in this error.

In general, data needs for PRA increase when $p[x, z]$ varies in time and/or space. Such variation is common in environmental and ecological science (Astigarraga et al., 2020). For example, climate change implies change in $p[x]$, and any adjustment of vegetation management, age structure or genetic composition affects the vulnerability of ecosystems to their environment (as represented by $p[z|x]$). Proper modelling of changes in $p[x]$ can benefit from open access to modelled predictions of climate change (e.g. https://www.metoffice.gov.uk/services/data). Data that quantify variation in vulnerability of ecosystems to environmental hazards are likely to be more critical.

Our spatial example focused on drought risk to forests in Scotland. Many studies on the impact of drought on forests have been published (e.g. Albrich et al., 2020, Anderegg et al., 2020, Cailleret et al., 2020, Davies et al., 2020, García-Valdés et al., 2020, Han and Singh, 2020, Lecina-Diaz et al., 2020, Pappas et al., 2020, Paschalis et al., 2020, Sharma and Panu, 2012, Thrippleton et al., 2020, and Trotsiuk et al., 2020) albeit without any formal risk analysis as developed here. Robust modelling of the vulnerability of trees to drought is hampered by incomplete knowledge and quantification of the underlying mechanisms (Eckes-Shephard et al., 2021; Mackay et al., 2020; McDowell et al., 2020; Wiley, 2020; Zellweger et al., 2020).

Sampling-based PRA, as developed here, has minimal computational demand. Distribution- and model-based PRA, on the other hand, require the use of Monte Carlo methods and thus are unsuitable for any real-time online calculation. Some speed-up of distribution-based PRA is possible by using the approximations for the integrals $E[z|x < thr]$ and $E[z|x \geq thr]$ that we presented in Chaps. 2 and 4.

However, these approximations rely on the assumption of normality for $p[x, z]$ and thus are unlikely to be commonly applicable.

19.3 BDT

For every decision-problem, BDT is optimal in the obvious sense that it identifies the action for which utility-expectation is maximised. However, this assumes an agreed-upon utility function. In practice, that agreement is not always present and the consequent value ambiguity may hamper the applicability of BDT (Lindley, 2000; Sahlin et al., 2021). Nevertheless, the implementation of BDT using Bayesian networks does facilitate stakeholder involvement. This has been demonstrated in environmental management (Gonzalez-Redin et al., 2016; Smith et al., 2012) where people were invited to co-design the network by discussing the variables and influences that the graph needed to represent. The discussions focused on elucidating *causal* pathways which kept the graphs sparse and understandable (Van Oijen, 2020 Chap. 15). Krich et al. (2020) presented a graph-based method for identifying causal links between environmental and ecosystem variables.

The graphical model of Fig. 12.1 showed the key elements and relationships of decision problems. A simple realisation of the graphical model was our toy example for BDT that we studied in Fig. 12.3. In this toy model, the degree of uncertainty affected the value of the optimum action. This effect of uncertainty is common in decision-making. For example, Tibshirani et al. (2011) showed that the optimum target for a darts-thrower to aim at depends on the precision with which they can throw the darts.

There are always three options concerning a specific action a: (1) decide to do a, (2) decide not to do a, (3) do not decide for or against a but decide to get more information first. The latter option is formally handled in BDT through the concept of *Value of Information* (VoI) which is the expected gain in utility if uncertainties are partly or wholly resolved through measurement before actions are decided upon (Lindley, 1991; Van Oijen, 2020, Chap. 17). We may want to examine the benefit from reducing uncertainties in model predictions before using them in decision-support. Li et al. (2017) showed how multiple models for Ebola could best be used together in decision-making. They ranked uncertainties using the VoI and showed that the models differed little in their identification of best disease management despite large variation in caseload prediction.

Management is a continuous process: new decisions will always have to be made at future dates. Fortunately, monitoring of ecosystems and of the consequences of the decisions will keep providing information that can be used to reduce parameter and driver uncertainties. Bayes' Theorem—which is of course intrinsic to BDT—is the tool with which the uncertainty reduction is calculated to make future decisions better informed. This continuous-learning aspect of Bayesian methods poses no conceptual problems, but it does mean that the efficiency and speed with which the information is processed is of major importance (Dorazio & Johnson, 2003).

19.4 Computational Demand of BDT

The computational demand of BDT is high because of (1) the double iteration: over parameter uncertainty and action choice, (2) the complexity of the Bayesian Hierarchical Model implied by the graphical model, (3) the complexity of any process-based models used (Van Oijen, 2020 Chap. 9), (4) requirements to repeat calculations over space and time (Lin et al., 1999; Timonina-Farkas et al., 2015; Trevisani, 2005). To mitigate these problems, we may want to replace the full calculations at least partly by PRA (leading to what we might call 'Approximate Bayesian Computation Decision Theory' or ABCDT). A more obvious approach would be to use emulators, not only for any process-based models (PBMs) but also for utility itself. This would make the BDT akin to a kriging exercise. The double iteration, which involves the need to run an MCMC for each evaluated action level, may benefit from parallel processing.

We showed how a simple Gaussian Process emulator could be derived from limited knowledge of model input-output relations, and that in many cases (i.e. grid cells in our spatial example for Scotland) the emulator produces the same output values as the original model, albeit with extra uncertainty. We did find that the emulator was unreliable when applied to grid cells with extreme environmental conditions. This is likely a general problem with emulators: they may not fully capture the nonlinear behaviour of the original model, and nonlinearity tends to be greatest near the extremes of the model-input domain. Moreover, extreme conditions are likely to be those for which measurements are scarce, so the to-be-emulated model itself may be least reliable for such conditions. In such cases, it is important to analyse the sensitivity of action selection to model assumptions and parameterisation.

19.5 PRA as a Tool for Simplifying and Elucidating BDT

The BDT provides a general approach to decision-making under uncertainty whereas the PRA just focuses on one element in the decision problem, namely the decomposition of risk posed by a hazard to system performance. When providing information to decision-makers, the full BDT approach may be hard to convey, and the PRA may play a useful role. The BDT defines the optimum action as the one that maximises expected utility, and we could use PRA to compare two or three actions (e.g. the optimal one according to BDT, 'business-as-usual,' and 'do-nothing'). For those actions the PRA could compare the hazard probabilities and the system vulnerabilities. This could be done at two levels: system performance y and utility u. A possible outcome of this approach could be: "We identified action a_{opt} as the best one, and it is superior to doing nothing because it reduces system vulnerability to the hazard by 20%." We could extend this by analysing how the environmental conditions x affect system vulnerability. Typically, x is multivariate so we may want to know, for example, which soil conditions predispose forests to drought vulnerability.

We showed that our spatial problem could be tackled in two equivalent ways: maximising the expectation for utility $E[U]$ or minimising the *corrected risk* R_c. Both methods showed that—for our example model—irrigation would only be advisable in eastern coastal regions of Scotland. One advantage of choosing to take the PRA-route is that it not only produces a map for the R_c but also gives us maps for $p[H]$, V, and R. Figure 17.3 shows the risk-components which make clear that where irrigation is required, it is due to high $p[H]$ and not high V.

19.6 Parameter and Model Uncertainties

In the earlier chapters, we discussed parameter uncertainties at length, but in some of our later examples we ignored that type of uncertainty. In practical problems, all uncertainties must be accounted for, but that would not affect our R-code chunks in a major way, except for the need to replace deterministic functions with sampling-based numerical integration when we calculate $E[U]$.

Likewise, we ignored model structural uncertainties, which is a more difficult problem. We may want to include uncertainty about model error (i.e. discrepancy) explicitly or use ensembles of models (Van Oijen, 2020, Chaps. 12–13). As an example of this from another field, Shea et al. (2020) discuss how the availability of multiple models, with different strengths and weaknesses, can be used to quantify uncertainties in a decision-theoretical approach to managing responses to epidemics.

19.7 Modelling and Decision-Support for Forest Response to Hazards

In this book, we used a very simple example of forest irrigation to explore algorithms for PRA and BDT. In practice, forests are subject to more hazards than just drought, possible actions involve more than irrigation (Holl & Brancalion, 2020), and benefits extend beyond forest productivity. Decision support systems must reconcile the many different conflicting demands on forests (Rauscher, 1999; Reynolds et al., 2017). Nevertheless, as in our example, there is always the requirement to define a utility-function that quantifies the balance of costs and benefits. This means that our code examples will need to be made more detailed for practical application, but not much more complex.

This also applies to the forest productivity model that we used, which in practice may need to be replaced by more complicated process-based models (PBMs). To run such models, more detailed data are required than just maps of altitude and precipitation. However, despite their apparent complexity, PBMs are still mathematical functions that map inputs to outputs, and they can be used in the same way in PRA and BDT as our simple one-line model was here. Anderegg et al. (2020) review the literature on measuring and modelling the impacts of climate extremes on forests and find that knowledge of drought impacts on forests are generally well implemented in PBMs, and they call for stronger inclusion of the models in decision-making. However, simpler models still dominate. For example, Davies et al. (2020) use the ESC decision-support system with look-up tables to assess future drought risk to 20 forest timber tree species in Scotland.

19.8   Spatial Statistics

Our example decision problem was spatial in the sense that we wanted to decide where in Scotland irrigation would be advisable. But most of our calculations were carried out separately for each grid cell on the basis of its local altitude and time series of precipitation. Only the extension to calculation of regional *exposure* to drought was a step toward spatial statistics. This is no problem when spatially consistent input data are available, such as the WorldClim maps of precipitation for 2000–2018. But if we want to employ PRA or BDT for future conditions, we must be wary of analysing each cell independently, because weather conditions are correlated in space (Timonina-Farkas et al., 2013). As Timonina-Farkas et al. (2015) states: "Hazards typically spread over wider areas. Hence, risk assessment must take into account interrelations between regions. Neglecting such dependencies can lead to a severe underestimation of potential losses, especially for extreme events." Future exposure cannot be assessed accurately without accounting for spatial correlations.

References

Albrich, K., Rammer, W., Turner, M.G., Ratajczak, Z., Braziunas, K.H., Hansen, W.D., & Seidl, R. (2020). Simulating forest resilience: A review. *Global Ecology and Biogeography, 29*, 2082–2096. https://doi.org/10.1111/geb.13197

Anderegg, W.R.L., Trugman, A.T., Badgley, G., Anderson, C.M., Bartuska, A., Ciais, P., Cullenward, D., Field, C.B., Freeman, J., Goetz, S.J., Hicke, J.A., Huntzinger, D., Jackson, R.B., Nickerson, J., Pacala, S., & Randerson, J.T. (2020). Climate-driven risks to the climate mitigation potential of forests. *Science, 368*. https://doi.org/10.1126/science.aaz7005

Astigarraga, J., Andivia, E., Zavala, M.A., Gazol, A., Cruz-Alonso, V., Vicente-Serrano, S.M., & Ruiz-Benito, P. (2020). Evidence of non-stationary relationships between climate and forest responses: Increased sensitivity to climate change in Iberian forests. *Global Change Biology, 26*, 5063–5076. https://doi.org/10.1111/gcb.15198

Bayes, T., 1763. An essay towards solving a problem in the doctrine of chances. *Philosophical Transactions, 53*, 370–418. https://doi.org/10.1098/rstl.1763.0053

Bedford, T., & Cooke, R. (2001). *Probabilistic risk analysis: Foundations and methods*. Cambridge University Press.

Berger, J.O. (1985). *Statistical decision theory and bayesian analysis* (2nd. ed.). *Springer series in statistics*. Springer-Verlag.

Bordley, R.F., & Pollock, S.M. (2009). A decision-analytic approach to reliability-based design optimization. *Operations Research, 57*, 1262–1270. https://doi.org/10.1287/opre.1080.0661

Borghetti, M., Gentilesca, T., Colangelo, M., Ripullone, F., & Rita, A. (2020). Xylem functional traits as indicators of health in mediterranean forests. *Current Forestry Reports, 6*, 220–236. https://doi.org/10.1007/s40725-020-00124-5

Borgonovo, E., Cappelli, V., Maccheroni, F., & Marinacci, M. (2018). Risk analysis and decision theory: A bridge. *European Journal of Operational Research, 264*, 280–293. https://doi.org/10.1016/j.ejor.2017.06.059

Brodribb, T.J., Powers, J., Cochard, H., & Choat, B. (2020). Hanging by a thread? Forests and drought. *Science, 368*, 261–266. https://doi.org/10.1126/science.aat7631

Brun, P., Psomas, A., Ginzler, C., Thuiller, W., Zappa, M., & Zimmermann, N.E. (2020). Large-scale early-wilting response of Central European forests to the 2018 extreme drought. *Global Change Biology, 26*, 7021–7035. https://doi.org/10.1111/gcb.15360

Butler, A., Heffernan, J.E., Tawn, J.A., Flather, R.A., & Horsburgh, K.J. (2007). Extreme value analysis of decadal variations in storm surge elevations. *Journal of Marine Systems, 67*, 189–200. https://doi.org/10.1016/j.jmarsys.2006.10.006

© The Author(s), under exclusive license to Springer Nature Switzerland AG 2022
M. van Oijen, M. Brewer, *Probabilistic Risk Analysis and Bayesian Decision Theory*, SpringerBriefs in Statistics, https://doi.org/10.1007/978-3-031-16333-3

Cailleret, M., Bircher, N., Hartig, F., Hülsmann, L., & Bugmann, H. (2020). Bayesian calibration of a growth-dependent tree mortality model to simulate the dynamics of European temperate forests. *Ecological Applications, 30*, e02021. https://doi.org/10.1002/eap.2021

Castillo, E., Menéndez, J.M., & Sánchez-Cambronero, S. (2008). Predicting traffic flow using Bayesian networks. *Transportation Research Part B: Methodological, 42*, 482–509. https://doi.org/10.1016/j.trb.2007.10.003

Cox, L.A., Jr. (2008). What's wrong with risk matrices? *Risk Analysis, 28*, 497–512. https://doi.org/10.1111/j.1539-6924.2008.01030.x

Davies, S., Bathgate, S., Petr, M., Gale, A., Patenaude, G., & Perks, M. (2020). Drought risk to timber production: A risk versus return comparison of commercial conifer species in Scotland. *Forest Policy and Economics, 117*, 102189. https://doi.org/10.1016/j.forpol.2020.102189

Dorazio, R.M., & Johnson, F.A. (2003). Bayesian inference and decision theory: A framework for decision making in natural resource management. *Ecological Applications, 13*, 556–563. https://doi.org/10.1890/1051-0761(2003)013%5B0556:BIADTA%5D2.0.CO;2

Eckes-Shephard, A.H., Tiavlovsky, E., Chen, Y., Fonti, P., & Friend, A.D. (2021). Direct response of tree growth to soil water and its implications for terrestrial carbon cycle modelling. *Global Change Biology, 27*, 121–135. https://doi.org/10.1111/gcb.15397

Embrechts, P., Lindskog, F., & Mcneil, A. (2003). Modelling dependence with copulas and applications to risk management. In *Handbook of heavy tailed distributions in finance* (pp. 329–384). Elsevier. https://doi.org/10.1016/B978-044450896-6.50010-8

Field, C.B., Barros, V., Stocker, T.F., & Dahe, Q. (Eds.) (2012). *Managing the risks of extreme events and disasters to advance climate change adaptation: Special report of the intergovernmental panel on climate change.* Cambridge University Press.

García-Valdés, R., Estrada, A., Early, R., Lehsten, V., & Morin, X. (2020). Climate change impacts on long-term forest productivity might be driven by species turnover rather than by changes in tree growth. *Global Ecology and Biogeography, 29*, 1360–1372. https://doi.org/10.1111/geb.13112

Genest, C., & Favre, A.-C. (2007). Everything you always wanted to know about copula modeling but were afraid to ask. *Journal of Hydrologic Engineering, 12*, 347–368. https://doi.org/10.1061/(ASCE)1084-0699(2007)12:4(347)

Gessler, A., Bottero, A., Marshall, J., & Arend, M. (2020). The way back: Recovery of trees from drought and its implication for acclimation. *New Phytologist, 228*(6), 1704–1709. https://doi.org/10.1111/nph.16703

Gonzalez-Redin, J., Luque, S., Poggio, L., Smith, R., & Gimona, A. (2016). Spatial Bayesian belief networks as a planning decision tool for mapping ecosystem services trade-offs on forested landscapes. *Environmental Research, The Provision of Ecosystem Services in Response to Global Change, 144*, 15–26. https://doi.org/10.1016/j.envres.2015.11.009

Guérin, M., von Arx, G., Martin-Benito, D., Andreu-Hayles, L., Griffin, K.L., McDowell, N.G., Pockman, W., & Gentine, P. (2020). Distinct xylem responses to acute vs prolonged drought in pine trees. *Tree Physiology, 40*, 605–620. https://doi.org/10.1093/treephys/tpz144

Han, J., & Singh, V.P. (2020). Forecasting of droughts and tree mortality under global warming: A review of causative mechanisms and modeling methods. *Journal of Water and Climate Change, 11*, 600–632. https://doi.org/10.2166/wcc.2020.239

Hao, Z., Hao, F., Singh, V.P., Ouyang, W., Zhang, X., & Zhang, S. (2020). A joint extreme index for compound droughts and hot extremes. *Theoretical and Applied Climatology, 142*, 321–328. https://doi.org/10.1007/s00704-020-03317-x

He, Q., Ju, W., Dai, S., He, W., Song, L., Wang, S., Li, X., & Mao, G. (2021). Drought risk of global terrestrial gross primary productivity over the last 40 years detected by a remote sensing-driven process model. *Journal of Geophysical Research: Biogeosciences, 126*. https://doi.org/10.1029/2020JG005944

HM_Government (2020). *National risk register.* https://www.gov.uk/government/publications/national-risk-register-2020

Hofert, M., Kojadinovic, I., Maechler, M., Yan, J., Nešlehová, J.G., & Morger, R. (2020). *Copula: Multivariate dependence with copulas.* https://CRAN.R-project.org/package=copula.

Holl, K.D., & Brancalion, P.H.S. (2020). Tree planting is not a simple solution. *Science, 368*, 580–581. https://doi.org/10.1126/science.aba8232

Huard, D., Évin, G., & Favre, A.-C. (2006). Bayesian copula selection. *Computational Statistics & Data Analysis, 51*(2), 809–822. https://doi.org/10.1016/j.csda.2005.08.010

Ionescu, C., Klein, R.J.T., Hinkel, J., Kavi Kumar, K.S., & Klein, R. (2009). Towards a formal framework of vulnerability to climate change. *Environmental Modeling & Assessment, 14*, 1–16. https://doi.org/10.1007/s10666-008-9179-x

IPCC (2014). *AR5 climate change 2014: Impacts, adaptation, and vulnerability*. Annex II - Glossary.

Jane, R.A., Simmonds, D.J., Gouldby, B.P., Simm, J.D., Valle, L.D., & Raby, A.C. (2018). Exploring the potential for multivariate fragility representations to alter flood risk estimates. *Risk Analysis, 38*, 1847–1870. https://doi.org/10.1111/risa.13007

Kannenberg, S.A., Schwalm, C.R., & Anderegg, W.R.L. (2020). Ghosts of the past: How drought legacy effects shape forest functioning and carbon cycling. *Ecology Letters, 23*, 891–901. https://doi.org/10.1111/ele.13485

Kaplan, S., & Garrick, B.J. (1981). On the quantitative definition of risk. *Risk Analysis, 1*, 11–27.

Khan, F.I., Amyotte, P.R., & Amin, M.T. (2020). Advanced methods of risk assessment and management: An overview. In F.I. Khan, & P.R. Amyotte (Eds.), *Methods in chemical process safety* (pp. 1–34). *Advanced Methods of Risk Assessment and Management*. Elsevier. https://doi.org/10.1016/bs.mcps.2020.03.002

Khoury, S., & Coomes, D.A. (2020). Resilience of Spanish forests to recent droughts and climate change. *Global Change Biology, 26*, 7079–7098. https://doi.org/10.1111/gcb.15268

Krich, C., Runge, J., Miralles, D.G., Migliavacca, M., Perez-Priego, O., El-Madany, T., Carrara, A., & Mahecha, M.D. (2020). Estimating causal networks in biosphereatmosphere interaction with the PCMCI approach. *Biogeosciences, 17*, 1033–1061. https://doi.org/10.5194/bg-17-1033-2020

Kuhnert, M., Yeluripati, J., Smith, P., Hoffmann, H., Van Oijen, M., Constantin, J., Dechow, R., Eckersten, H., Gaiser, T., Grosz, B., Haas, E., Kersebaum, K.-C., Kiese, R., Klatt, S., Lewan, E., Nendel, C., Raynal, H., Sosa, C., Specka, X., Teixeira, E., Wang, E., Weihermüller, L., Zhao, G., Zhao, Z., Ogle, & Ewert, F. (2017). Impact analysis of climate data aggregation at different spatial scales on simulated net primary productivity for croplands. *European Journal of Agronomy, 88*, 41–52.

Laux, P., Vogl, S., Qiu, W., Knoche, H.R., & Kunstmann, H. (2011). Copula-based statistical refinement of precipitation in RCM simulations over complex terrain. *Hydrology and Earth System Sciences, 15*, 2401–2419. https://doi.org/10.5194/hess-15-2401-2011

Lecina-Diaz, J., Martínez-Vilalta, J., Alvarez, A., Banqué, M., Birkmann, J., Feldmeyer, D., Vayreda, J., & Retana, J. (2020). Characterizing forest vulnerability and risk to climate-change hazards. *Frontiers in Ecology and the Environment, 19*(3), 126–133. https://doi.org/10.1002/fee.2278

Li, S.-L., Bjørnstad, O.N., Ferrari, M.J., Mummah, R., Runge, M.C., Fonnesbeck, C.J., Tildesley, M.J., Probert, W.J.M., & Shea, K. (2017). Essential information: Uncertainty and optimal control of Ebola outbreaks. *Proceedings of the National Academy of Sciences of the United States of America, 114*, 5659–5664. https://doi.org/10.1073/pnas.1617482114

Li, Y., Dong, & Y., Zhu, D. (2020). Copula-based vulnerability analysis of civil infrastructure subjected to hurricanes. *Frontiers in Built Environment, 6*, 571911. https://doi.org/10.3389/fbuil.2020.571911

Lin, C., Gelman, A., Price, P.N., & Krantz, D.H. (1999). Analysis of local decisions using hierarchical modeling, applied to home radon measurement and remediation. *Statistical Science, 14*, 305–337. https://doi.org/10.1214/ss/1009212411

Lindley, D.V. (2000). The philosophy of statistics. *Journal of the Royal Statistical Society. Series D (The Statistician), 49*, 293–337.

Lindley, D.V. (1991). *Making decisions* (2nd ed.). John Wiley & Sons.

Mackay, D.S., Savoy, P.R., Grossiord, C., Tai, X., Pleban, J.R., Wang, D.R., McDowell, N.G., Adams, H.D., & Sperry, J.S. (2020). Conifers depend on established roots during drought:

Results from a coupled model of carbon allocation and hydraulics. *New Phytologist, 225*, 679–692. https://doi.org/10.1111/nph.16043

Mazumder, A. (2003). Statistical decision theory concepts, methods and applications. Special topics in Probabilistic Graphical Models. Wiley.

McDowell, N.G., Allen, C.D., Anderson-Teixeira, K., Aukema, B.H., Bond-Lamberty, B., Chini, L., Clark, J.S., Dietze, M., Grossiord, C., Hanbury-Brown, A., Hurtt, G.C., Jackson, R.B., Johnson, D.J., Kueppers, L., Lichstein, J.W., Ogle, K., Poulter, B., Pugh, T.A.M., Seidl, R., Turner, M.G., Uriarte, M., Walker, A.P., & Xu, C., 2020. Pervasive shifts in forest dynamics in a changing world. *Science, 368*. https://doi.org/10.1126/science.aaz9463

Mee, R.W., & Owen, D.B. (1983). A simple approximation for bivariate normal probabilities. *Journal of Quality Technology, 15*, 72–75. https://doi.org/10.1080/00224065.1983.11978848

Nandintsetseg, B., Boldgiv, B., Chang, J., Ciais, P., Davaanyam, E., Batbold, A., Bat-Oyun, T., & Stenseth, N.C. (2021). Risk and vulnerability of Mongolian grasslands under climate change. *Environmental Research Letters, 16*, 034035. https://doi.org/10.1088/1748-9326/abdb5b

Nelsen, R.B. (2007). *An introduction to copulas* (2nd ed.). Springer.

Nguyen-Huy, T., Deo, R.C., Mushtaq, S., Kath, J., & Khan, S. (2018). Copula-based agricultural conditional value-at-risk modelling for geographical diversifications in wheat farming portfolio management. *Weather and Climate Extremes, 21*, 76–89. https://doi.org/10.1016/j.wace.2018.07.002

Pappas, C., Peters, R.L., & Fonti, P. (2020). Linking variability of tree water use and growth with species resilience to environmental changes. *Ecography, 43*(9), 1386–1399. https://doi.org/10.1111/ecog.04968

Parmigiani, G., & Inoue, L.Y.T. (2009). *Decision theory: Principles and approaches*. Wiley.

Paschalis, A., Fatichi, S., Zscheischler, J., Ciais, P., Bahn, M., Boysen, L., Chang, J., Kauwe, M.D., Estiarte, M., Goll, D., Hanson, P.J., Harper, A.B., Hou, E., Kigel, J., Knapp, A.K., Larsen, K.S., Li, W., Lienert, S., Luo, Y., Meir, P., Nabel, J.E.M.S., Ogaya, R., Parolari, A.J., Peng, C., Peñuelas, J., Pongratz, J., Rambal, S., Schmidt, I.K., Shi, H., Sternberg, M., Tian, H., Tschumi, E., Ukkola, A., Vicca, S., Viovy, N., Wang, Y.-P., Wang, Z., Williams, K., Wu, D., & Zhu, Q. (2020). Rainfall manipulation experiments as simulated by terrestrial biosphere models: Where do we stand? *Global Change Biology, 26*, 3336–3355. https://doi.org/10.1111/gcb.15024

Rausand, M. (2020). *Risk assessment: Theory, methods, and applications* (1st ed.). Wiley. https://doi.org/10.1002/9781119377351

Rauscher, H.M. (1999). Ecosystem management decision support for federal forests in the United States: A review. *Forest Ecology and Management, 114*, 173–197. https://doi.org/10.1016/0378-1127(76)90002-5

Reynolds, K.M., Murphy, P.J., & Paplanus, S. (2017). Toward geodesign for watershed restoration on the fremont-winema national forest, Pacific Northwest, USA. *Sustainability, 9*, 678. https://doi.org/10.3390/su9050678

Rosen, O., & Thompson, W.K. (2015). Bayesian semiparametric copula estimation with application to psychiatric genetics: Bayesian semiparametric copula estimation. *Biometrical Journal, 57*, 468–484. https://doi.org/10.1002/bimj.201300130

Sahlin, U., Troffaes, M.C.M., & Edsman, L. (2021). Robust decision analysis under severe uncertainty and ambiguous tradeoffs: An invasive species case study. arXiv:2103.04721 [stat].

Salvadori, G., Durante, F., De Michele, C., & Bernardi, M. (2018). Hazard assessment under multivariate distributional change-points: Guidelines and a flood case study. *Water, 10*, 751. https://doi.org/10.3390/w10060751

Schölzel, C., & Friederichs, P. (2008). Multivariate non-normally distributed random variables in climate research introduction to the copula approach. *Nonlinear Processes in Geophysics, 15*, 761–772. https://doi.org/10.5194/npg-15-761-2008

Schuldt, B., Buras, A., Arend, M., Vitasse, Y., Beierkuhnlein, C., Damm, A., Gharun, M., Grams, T.E.E., Hauck, M., Hajek, P., Hartmann, H., Hiltbrunner, E., Hoch, G., Holloway-Phillips, M., Körner, C., Larysch, E., Lübbe, T., Nelson, D.B., Rammig, A., Rigling, A., Rose, L., Ruehr, N.K., Schumann, K., Weiser, F., Werner, C., Wohlgemuth, T., Zang, C.S., & Kahmen, A. (2020). A first assessment of the impact of the extreme 2018 summer drought on Central

European forests. *Basic and Applied Ecology, 45*, 86–103. https://doi.org/10.1016/j.baae.2020. 04.003

Serinaldi, F., Lombardo, F., & Kilsby, C.G. (2020). All in order: Distribution of serially correlated order statistics with applications to hydrological extremes. *Advances in Water Resources, 144*, 103686. https://doi.org/10.1016/j.advwatres.2020.103686

Shachter, R.D., & Kenley, C.R. (1989). Gaussian influence diagrams. *Management Science, 35*, 527–550. https://doi.org/10.1287/mnsc.35.5.527

Sharma, T.C., & Panu, U.S. (2012). Prediction of hydrological drought durations based on Markov chains: Case of the Canadian prairies. *Hydrological Sciences Journal, 57*, 705–722. https://doi. org/10.1080/02626667.2012.672741

Shea, K., Runge, M.C., Pannell, D., Probert, W.J.M., Li, S.-L., Tildesley, M., & Ferrari, M. (2020). Harnessing multiple models for outbreak management. *Science, 368*, 577–579. https://doi.org/ 10.1126/science.abb9934

Shen, W., Tokdar, S.T., & Ghosal, S. (2013). Adaptive Bayesian multivariate density estimation with Dirichlet mixtures. *Biometrika, 100*, 623–640. https://doi.org/10.1093/biomet/ast015

Smith, R., Dick, J., Trench, H., & Van Oijen, M. (2012). Extending a Bayesian belief network for ecosystem evaluation. In *Conference paper of the 2012 Berlin conference of the human dimensions of global environmental change on evidence for sustainable development, 5–6 October 2012, Berlin, Germany.*

Szejner, P., Belmecheri, S., Ehleringer, J.R., & Monson, R.K. (2020). Recent increases in drought frequency cause observed multi-year drought legacies in the tree rings of semi-arid forests. *Oecologia, 192*, 241–259. https://doi.org/10.1007/s00442-019-04550-6

Thomas, P., Bratvold, R.B., & Eric, B.J. (2014). The risk of using risk matrices. *SPE Economics and Management, April 2014*, D011S007R003. https://doi.org/10.2118/166269-MS

Thrippleton, T., Hülsmann, L., Cailleret, M., & Bugmann, H. (2020). Projecting forest dynamics across Europe: Potentials and pitfalls of empirical mortality algorithms. *Ecosystems, 23*, 188–203. https://doi.org/10.1007/s10021-019-00397-3

Tibshirani, R.J., Price, A., & Taylor, J. (2011). A statistician plays darts. *Journal of the Royal Statistical Society: Series A (Statistics in Society), 174*, 213–226. https://doi.org/10.1111/j. 1467-985X.2010.00651.x

Timonina-Farkas, A., Hochrainer-Stigler, S., Pflug, G., Jongman, B., & Rojas, R. (2015). Structured coupling of probability loss distributions: Assessing joint flood risk in multiple river basins. *Risk Analysis, 35*, 2102–2119.

Timonina-Farkas, A., Mechler, R., Williges, K., & Hochrainer-Stigler, S. (2013). *Catalogue and Toolbox of risk assessment and management tools.* Deliverable 2.1. ENHANCE.

Trevisani, M. (2005) Bayesian decision models for environmental risks. In *S.I.S. 2005 - Statistica e Ambiente* (pp. 21–23) September 2005, Messina, Italy.

Trotsiuk, V., Hartig, F., Cailleret, M., Babst, F., Forrester, D.I., Baltensweiler, A., Buchmann, N., Bugmann, H., Gessler, A., Gharun, M., Minunno, F., Rigling, A., Rohner, B., Stillhard, J., Thürig, E., Waldner, P., Ferretti, M., Eugster, W., & Schaub, M. (2020). Assessing the response of forest productivity to climate extremes in Switzerland using modeldata fusion. *Global Change Biology, 26*(4), 2463–2476. https://doi.org/10.1111/gcb.15011

UN. (1992). *Internationally agreed glossary of basic terms related to disaster management.* Department of Humanitarian Affairs.

Van Oijen, M. (2020). *Bayesian compendium.* Springer International Publishing. https://doi.org/ 10.1007/978-3-030-55897-0

Van Oijen, M., Balkovic, J., Beer, C., Cameron, D.R., Ciais, P., Cramer, W., Kato, T., Kuhnert, M., Martin, R., Myneni, R., Rammig, A., Rolinski, S., Soussana, J.-F., Thonicke, K., Van der Velde, M., & Xu, L. (2014). Impact of droughts on the carbon cycle in European vegetation: A probabilistic risk analysis using six vegetation models. *Biogeosciences, 11*, 6357–6375. https:// doi.org/10.5194/bg-11-6357-2014

Van Oijen, M., Beer, C., Cramer, W., Rammig, A., Reichstein, M., Rolinski, S., & Soussana, J.-F. (2013). A novel probabilistic risk analysis to determine the vulnerability of ecosystems to extreme climatic events. *Environmental Research Letters, 8*, 015032. https://doi.org/10.1088/1748-9326/8/1/015032

Van Oijen, M., & Zavala, M.A. (2019). Probabilistic drought risk analysis for even-aged forests. In J. Sillmann, S. Sippel, & S. Russo (Eds.), Climate extremes and their implications for impact and risk assessment (pp. 159–176). Elsevier.

Vehtari, A., & Ojanen, J. (2012). A survey of Bayesian predictive methods for model assessment, selection and comparison. *Statistics Surveys, 6*, 142–228. https://doi.org/10.1214/12-SS102

Venäläinen, A., Lehtonen, I., Laapas, M., Ruosteenoja, K., Tikkanen, O.-P., Viiri, H., Ikonen, V.-P., & Peltola, H. (2020). Climate change induces multiple risks to boreal forests and forestry in Finland: A literature review. *Global Change Biology, 26*, 4178–4196. https://doi.org/10.1111/gcb.15183

Villar-Hernández, B. de J., Pérez-Elizalde, S., Crossa, J., Pérez-Rodríguez, P., Toledo, F.H., & Burgueño, J. (2018). A Bayesian decision theory approach for genomic selection. *G3 Genes|Genomes|Genetics, 8*, 3019–3037. https://doi.org/10.1534/g3.118.200430

Wiley, E. (2020). Do carbon reserves increase tree survival during stress and following disturbance? *Current Forestry Reports, 6*, 14–25. https://doi.org/10.1007/s40725-019-00106-2

Williams, P.J., & Hooten, M.B. (2016). Combining statistical inference and decisions in ecology. *Ecological Applications, 26*, 1930–1942.

Zellweger, F., Frenne, P.D., Lenoir, J., Vangansbeke, P., Verheyen, K., Bernhardt-Römermann, M., Baeten, L., Hédl, R., Berki, I., Brunet, J., Calster, H.V., Chudomelová, M., Decocq, G., Dirnböck, T., Durak, T., Heinken, T., Jaroszewicz, B., Kopecký, M., Máliš, F., Macek, M., Malicki, M., Naaf, T., Nagel, T.A., Ortmann-Ajkai, A., Petřík, P., Pielech, R., Reczyńska, K., Schmidt, W., Standovár, T., Świerkosz, K., Teleki, B., Vild, O., Wulf, M., & Coomes, D. (2020). Response to Comment on "Forest microclimate dynamics drive plant responses to warming." *Science, 370*. https://doi.org/10.1126/science.abf2939

Zhou, L., Wang, S., Chi, Y., & Wang, J. (2018). Drought impacts on vegetation indices and productivity of terrestrial ecosystems in southwestern china during 2001. *Chinese Geographical Science, 28*, 784–796. https://doi.org/10.1007/s11769-018-0967-1

Zscheischler, J., Martius, O., Westra, S., Bevacqua, E., Raymond, C., Horton, R.M., van den Hurk, B., AghaKouchak, A., Jézéquel, A., Mahecha, M.D., Maraun, D., Ramos, A.M., Ridder, N.N., Thiery, W., & Vignotto, E. (2020). A typology of compound weather and climate events. *Nature Reviews Earth & Environment, 1*, 333–347. https://doi.org/10.1038/s43017-020-0060-z

Index

Printed in the United States
by Baker & Taylor Publisher Services